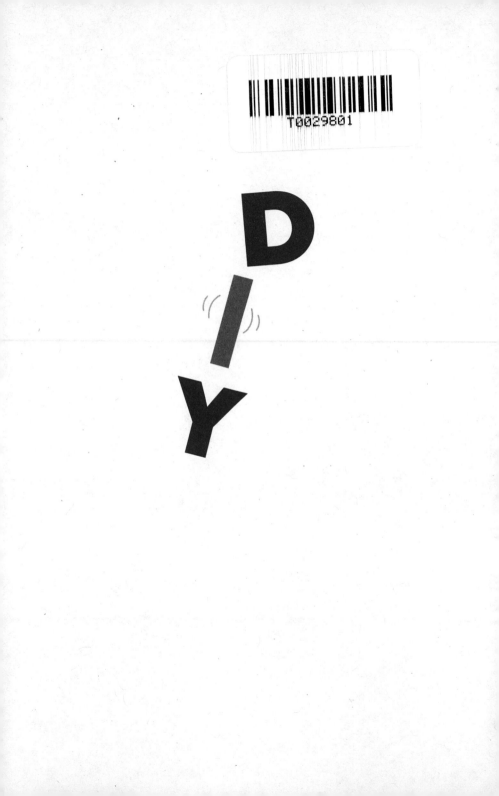

DIY

The Wonderfully
Weird History and
Science of
Masturbation

Dr. Eric Sprankle

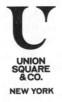

UNION
SQUARE
& CO.

NEW YORK

**UNION
SQUARE
& CO.**

NEW YORK

ISBN 978-1-4549-4879-7 (paperback)
ISBN 978-1-4549-4880-3 (e-book)

Library of Congress Control Number: 2023036761
Library of Congress Cataloging-in-Publication Data is available upon request.

For information about custom editions, special sales, and premium purchases, please
contact specialsales@unionsquareandco.com.

Printed in Canada

2 4 6 8 10 9 7 5 3 1

unionsquareandco.com

Cover design by Elizabeth Mihaltse Lindy
Interior design by Kevin Ullrich
Cover art by Shutterstock.com: buzzbee (right hand cover, back cover);
iced.espresso (left hand cover); ollikeballoon (bracelet)

For the bators and the haters

Contents

Introduction

Selling the Disease of Masturbation

D r. John Harvey Kellogg, a physician at the Battle Creek Sanitarium in Michigan in the late 1800s, was fixated on eradicating the "doubly abominable" act of masturbation. An act, he believed, to be the cause of many ailments among youth, including pimples, lusterless eyes, moist hands, uterine displacement, heart disease, tuberculosis, paralysis, and psychosis.

Assuming a diet of rich and spicy foods was a contributing factor in producing sexual desire, Dr. Kellogg sought to develop a bland food to dampen the sex drives of adolescents to steer them away from "self-pollution" and the "sin against nature." The result of his anti-masturbation crusade was the creation of Kellogg's Corn Flakes.[1] A cereal so bland, he hoped, that it would destroy penile and clitoral erections across the country.

Fortunately for those who enjoy masturbation and breakfast, Dr. Kellogg's cereal libido killer was based in pseudoscientific moralism. His Seventh-Day Adventist beliefs clouded his view of healthy sexuality, and his toasted corn flakes did not produce the desired effect on young people of late nineteenth-century America.

---

1. Although Dr. Kellogg held the original patent for his corn flakes, his brother, Will Kellogg, ultimately won the right to use the family name to form the Kellogg Company. After years of legal battles, Will Kellogg was free to sell the cereals and add lustful ingredients like sugar, paving the way for the sexual idolatry of Tony the Tiger.

It would be wonderful if this book was just focused on Dr. Kellogg, his contemporaries, and on the history of moral panic surrounding masturbation as some sort of relic of the past. You could giggle with your friends about all the ridiculous campaigns of yesteryear to suppress masturbation, which has included applying cold compresses to the spine and using enemas. You could wince at reading sadistic methods of eliminating masturbatory urges that included circumcising the foreskin without anesthesia and dousing the clitoris with carbolic acid. You could reflect on how fortunate it is to live in a time where that idiocy no longer exists.

But, unfortunately, we cannot have nice things.

Sexual progressiveness, from a historical perspective, is not a linear process. It has always been two orgasms forward, one orgasm back.

Masturbation of Yore

Much to Dr. Kellogg's chagrin, for most of human history, people masturbated without care or consequence. For thousands of years, we lived without the disapproving finger-waving from religious zealots, quacks, and wellness gurus trying to police what we do in the shadows with our own genitals.

Based on field observations of our closest primate relatives, *Pan paniscus*,[2] as well as other, more distantly related species like horses, porcupines, and walruses, masturbation is a common behavior within the animal kingdom. As such, there is no reason to believe early *Homo sapiens* would shy away from the pleasures of self-stimulation. However, according to psychology professor Dr. Jesse Bering, one key difference between human and nonhuman masturbation is that we are much more

---

2. Commonly known as bonobos, these apes are the hornier cousins of common chimpanzees and will often use sexual behaviors to defuse tension and conflict. They are regularly observed rubbing their carrot-like erections and enormously swollen vulvas with their hands, feet, and against objects, much to the amusement of onlooking families visiting wildlife sanctuaries.

likely to masturbate to orgasm instead of just diddling ourselves for a few moments before getting distracted by a passing squirrel.

Given our sizable cerebral cortex that allows for abstract thought, this brain structure also allows us to fantasize. Thus, we are able to create a sexually stimulating environment wherever we go and maintain this erotic world to climax. This gave our 42,000-year-old ancestors the ability to fantasize about that hunky Neanderthal seen earlier by the cave entrance, and the ability to masturbate to orgasm with phallic-shaped siltstone without any feelings of guilt or shame.

Thousands of years later, early human civilizations still paid little mind to masturbation as a destructive behavior. Void of any sense of immorality or unhealthiness tied to the practice, masturbation was often depicted in art and described in poetry, even among the gods. Greek philosopher Diogenes wrote in mythical jest that the god Hermes taught his son Pan (the half-man, half-goat frolicker) the practice of self-pleasure, and that he, in turn, could teach it to isolated shepherds tending to their flock.

And although the tolerance of masturbation in this time existed millennia before the emergence of medical hyperbole about "self-abuse," masturbation did begin to take its lowered place on the hierarchy of sexual appropriateness in polite society. The ancient Greeks viewed masturbation as the butt of jokes because the practice was reserved for those without a sexual partner. It was looked upon with pity—a last resort for someone's lonely genitals.

But being the butt of jokes aside, masturbation was also implicitly frowned upon for those of higher social status. It, along with many other sexual behaviors, was not viewed as a dignified behavior among the elites, but something those at the margins of civilized society (e.g., enslaved Persians, mythical satyrs) were expected to engage in because of their societal rank.

All of this changed with the dawn of *modern masturbation*. Not modern like dry humping a sex robot, but modern in that masturbation was re-contextualized as a disease of the modern age. In the 2003 academic tome *Solitary Sex: A Cultural History of Masturbation,* history professor Dr. Thomas Laqueur argues this re-contextualization began in the early eighteenth century when an anonymous pamphlet started circulating in parts of London warning about the physical dangers of masturbating. On par with the ridiculous claims within the pamphlet is the overly descriptive and inconsistently capitalized title: *Onania; or, The Heinous Sin of Self-Pollution, and all its Frightful Consequences, in both Sexes Considered, with Spiritual and Physical Advice to those who have already injured themselves by this abominable Practice. And seasonable Admonition to the Youth of the Nation, (of both Sexes) and those whose Tuition they are under, whether Parents, Guardians, Masters, or Mistresses.*

The pamphlet, costing anxious masturbators 1 shilling and 6 pence, sold tens of thousands of copies over the course of its oft-revised publication history within Europe's first mass media marketplace of booksellers. *Onania* was not short on repeating the talking points of priests and reverends who believed the devil whispers in your ear, trying to convince you that masturbating is harmless fun. Within the pamphlet's pages, masturbation was viewed as a gateway sin that will take the self-fondler down the path of lying, stealing, and murdering.

But what was new within *Onania* was its focus on the health effects, not just spiritual effects, of this "solitary vice." The anonymous author warned readers that masturbating would lead to fainting spells, melancholy, infertility, and epilepsy. For women, masturbation caused the skin's complexion to become "swarthy and hagged." For men, ejaculating was "robbing the body of its balmy and vital moisture" resulting in death, essentially arguing that ejaculation dehydrates you to the point of becoming a freeze-dried mummy.

The pseudoscientific moralism within *Onania* and its derivatives[3] struck a chord among western Europeans and Americans during the Enlightenment of the eighteenth century, where the values of freedom, autonomy, individualism, privacy, and imagination were challenging the oppressive political and religious regimes of the times. As such, reactionaries zeroed in on masturbation as a reflection of these values, believing, among other fallacies, that the biggest sin was having "an impure imagination." Tens of thousands of years earlier, this fantastical imagination of ours was setting us apart from other species. Now, pearl-clutching busybodies were explicitly condemning the use of our marvelous, sexually imaginative brains.

Digitally Masturbating

Despite these attitudes originating centuries ago, these are the anti-masturbation beliefs that persist today within the strange bedfellow circles of religious moralists, insecure misogynists, white supremacists, conservative politicians, and pseudoscientific health hucksters. The highly prevalent behavior of masturbation is still believed to be the destroyer of bodies, souls, and civilizations in the digital age.

Throughout this book, you will be introduced to the anti-masturbation crusaders who are trying to keep you from reaching into your pants. There are Christian pastors who are convinced Satan is preventing you from starting a family by encouraging you to masturbate.

---

3. Like Swiss physician Samuel–Auguste Tissot who published *L'Onanisme* in 1760 that warned of the physical dangers of masturbation and considered semen to be an "essential oil." The modern essential oil industry has yet to capitalize on this assertion by making semen diffusers for aromatherapy.

There are gym bros who believe ejaculating depletes your testosterone and muscle mass. There are white supremacists who encourage their fellow "genetically superior" brethren to abstain from self-pleasure in order to preserve the white race. There are legislators in the American South who support making it a crime to possess more than five sex toys, but who actively support citizens owning thirty-nine semi-automatic rifles (one for each conspiracy theory they believe). And there are Instagram wellness influencers who are unknowingly spreading the gospel of *Onania* by claiming that masturbation causes brain damage, depletes you of vital nutrients, and shrinks your penis.

But even though there are plenty of people and groups in the twenty-first century who are trying to protect you from the alleged harms of a self-induced orgasm, fortunately, there are hordes of others who are pushing back and liberating self-pleasure.

There are elementary school sex educators risking job security (and personal security) by teaching their students that it is normal to be curious about your body. There are university professors fighting to secure grant funding to better understand why those high in religiosity are more likely to believe they are addicted to masturbating. There are sex workers who navigate stigma, criminalization, de-platforming, and banking restrictions in order to masturbate in front of paying customers and clients. There are ingenious inventors who have created sex toys that can hold the cremated ashes of your deceased lover as a way to offer comfort to a grieving clitoris.

And between these two warring factions, the oppressors and the liberators, exists the majority of the population. The population for whom this book is written. The everyday person who is stuck in the middle of science and pseudoscience. The average Joe and Jane who just want to come home from work and come in peace without guilt and shame.

This book aims to serve as a guide to understanding sexual science as it pertains to masturbatory health.

The Modern Medicine Show

Writing a book solely devoted to debunking the myths associated with masturbation was never part of my academic five-year plan. It never crossed my mind that this book was needed. I assumed believing in hairy palms and blindness caused by masturbating died along with believing in the tooth fairy and American exceptionalism.

The modern-day Kelloggs proved me wrong.

I started receiving comments and messages on social media calling me unethical and irresponsible for saying masturbation is healthy. These accusers listed all the dangers of masturbating, like zinc loss, decreased gray matter in the brain, and depression. They were speaking with such authority and confidence that I assumed they had advance degrees in endocrinology, neuroscience, or psychiatry.

They did not.

But they did have blogs, YouTube channels, popular TikTok accounts, and unbridled arrogance. I marveled at their overconfidence in their own stupidity and wondered who would be gullible enough to believe in what they were ignorantly peddling. They reminded me of the traveling medicine shows of the nineteenth century, where grifters would attract audiences with wild and weird tales of diseases and then sell them a snake oil cure.

"Step right up, folks! Do you have gout? Cholera? Hemorrhoids? Then try Dr. Thornberry's Miracle Elixir, made from natural spring water, rose hips, and cocaine."

This modern masturbation medicine show dazzles audiences with the horrors of solitary sex and promises abstinence to be the panacea ushering in good health, loving relationships, financial success, and spiritual salvation. And while there are grifters among them selling subscriptions, personal coaching sessions, and detox programs, many are just gullible disciples sharing the gospel of self-denial to better manage their own sexual shame and insecurities.

When I first started pitching the idea of this book to literary agents and then to publishers, I struggled with articulating the type of book I envisioned that would best counter the internet misinformation about masturbation and that would be both scientifically literate and accessible to an average reader. It was challenging to clearly communicate how I wanted to combine health science, narrative, and prescriptive elements, all the while maintaining my oft-irreverent tone.

Although there is plenty of useful information in this book that can be applied to your personal sex life, I did not want to write a self-help book that was filled with oversimplified advice and hollow BuzzFeed-style lists like "10 Ways to Masturbate Like Your Favorite Lord of the Rings Character!"[4]

Although this book is heavily cited with peer-reviewed journal articles and other scholarly works, I did not want to write a serious academic book that was only sold at research conferences and was only entertaining to those who got aroused by effect sizes and p values. I wanted to write a book for a lay audience that is sold in mall bookstores where goth teens can intentionally place a copy in the Christian Romance section.

And although this book is peppered with historical accounts, I am not a historian or anthropologist. The historical descriptions will be brief and often superficial but used to drive a narrative that for the past three hundred years, for every Dr. Kellogg trying to scare you into sexual submission with grotesque fairy tales, there's been a Dr. Kinsey

---

4. Although this is a missed opportunity for a lot of Gandalf wizard staff jokes.

eager to alleviate your masturbatory anxieties with sexual science. For every Reverend Sylvester Graham trying to advocate for masturbation's suppression on moral grounds, there's a Betty Dodson advocating for its liberation.

This book exists at the intersection of all those genres. I'm here to tell you the story of the crusaders on a campaign to suppress masturbation, the sex educators fighting back, and the public's confusion about what constitutes healthy self-pleasure.

I will be your guide, walking you through these anti-masturbation medicine shows. Exploring topics such as normative behaviors during childhood, the NoFap and semen retention movements, the moral panic over masturbation addiction, dildos and sex dolls, porn and fantasy, and how death doulas are ensuring that masturbation can be a part of hospice care, this book aims to unapologetically critique the individuals and systems that have sought to control masturbation, and reviews the scientific literature and clinical recommendations on how masturbation is a healthy practice for all.

So, step right up, folks! Shudder at the thought of spiked penile rings used to prevent the solitary vice. Laugh at pastors who believe mermaids are created by the sin of self-pollution. Marvel at the ingenuity of a 28,000-year-old dildo. Grab a bowl of corn flakes and settle into a sofa to learn about the wonderfully weird history and science of masturbation. Worry-free orgasms await.

CHAPTER 1

Protect the Children

Child Development, Sex Education, and Masturbating Fetuses

I n 1994, the surgeon general of the United States, Dr. Joycelyn Elders, spoke to a group of sex educators and policy makers at a UNAIDS conference. During the Q&A session, a conference participant asked, "It seems to me that there still remains a taboo against the discussion about masturbation . . . I do want to ask you, what you think are the prospects [of] a more explicit discussion and promotion of masturbation?"

To which Dr. Elders replied, "As per your specific question in regard to masturbation, I think that is something that is a part of human sexuality and it's a part of something that perhaps should be taught. But we've not even taught our children the very basics. And I feel that we have tried ignorance for a very long time and it's time we try education."

It seems like a reasonable, off-the-cuff response, albeit a little tentative and avoidant, and certainly a far cry from explicitly and unequivocally supporting the topic of masturbation being included in sex education curriculum. But the reaction she received back in Washington, DC, was as if she supported teaching kids how to make Karl Marx dildos at a drag show.

President Bill Clinton was already trying to distance his administration from Dr. Elders and her previous comments on drug legalization,

DIY

harm-reduction approaches to support sex workers, and abortion.[5] Dr. Elders merely mentioning masturbation was the last straw for President Clinton, who wasn't exactly known for having a strong moral compass when it comes to sex. He felt the comments were different from his "own convictions" and so he fired her less than two weeks later.

Knee-jerk reactionaries like US Congressman Bob Dornan hailed the firing and took to the House floor earlier that year to declare that Dr. Elders "mocked American citizens who want public policy to reflect the Judeo-Christian ethical standards of our culture." For Representative Dornan and others who believe laws should reflect their personal religious beliefs, acknowledging the fact that young people touch their own genitals for pleasure is considered blasphemy. But masturbation is a reality for everyone, regardless of age and regardless of religion, and those claiming otherwise are projecting their own sexual fears, insecurities, and ignorance onto younger generations.

The Book of Genesis

In the beginning, we are floating around in a sack, unable to discern light from dark, and being sustained by a cord connected to a lump of cells. We hear nonsensical muffled sounds. We kick our generous host in the ribs at 2 a.m. We squeeze their bladder while they are stuck in traffic. We induce vomiting, swollen ankles, back pain, and hemorrhoids. We are a non-thinking, non-breathing bringer of chaos. And despite being in this primordial state, having just shed our tails a few weeks prior, we still engage in one of the few, near-universal joys of the human experience: We masturbate.

---

5. She once told the Catholic clergy to "get over their love affair with the fetus," which should have earned her the Presidential Medal of Freedom.

Although fetal masturbation is a topic usually avoided at baby showers and gender reveal parties, it does, nonetheless, exist as a reality for many developing organisms in the uterus. When I mention this fact at a dinner party, to which I will never be invited again, it is difficult for the other guests to comprehend. Apart from just wanting to eat their chicken and discuss their latest patio furniture purchase, the other diners struggle with understanding fetal masturbation because, like all of us, we are egocentric with sexuality. It is natural for us to believe our sexual thoughts, desires, motivations, and behaviors are shared by everyone. So, when we first learn about fetuses masturbating, we project our own experience of masturbation onto the fetus. We imagine it must be positioning its feet against the uterine wall and vigorously rubbing its underdeveloped genital lumps while fantasizing about the other fetuses from Lamaze class.

The reality for fetuses, however, is they lack the visual experience and neural development for memory to have sexual fantasies. They lack sufficient gonadal hormone production and the perception to experience anything remotely close to what we would consider sexual desire. But despite these sexuality shortcomings that adults take for granted, they do have enough manual dexterity to find their genitals and self-pleasure.

First documented by Dr. Israel Meizner in 1987 with an ultrasound of a twenty-eight-week-old fetus, the series of images showed repetitive hand movements on a grasped penis for several minutes. Follow-up studies by other researchers found similar results between eighteen and thirty-two weeks of gestation with penile stimulation that retracted the foreskin, clitoral rubbing to orgasm, and even penile sucking. Even in a larger study involving one hundred 2D ultrasound scans between eighteen and twenty-three weeks, 78 percent of the fetuses were observed masturbating. Anti-abortion activists are really missing out on a persuasive marketing opportunity by ignoring this research.

Infantile Gratification Phenomena

Infancy and early toddlerhood masturbation are very similar. Without the benefit of being suspended weightlessly in amniotic fluid, however, infants lose some manual dexterity for direct genital stimulation with their hands. As an alternative, they will cross their legs, arch their backs, and make sudden, writhing movements in order to self-stimulate. The movements are in conjunction with face-flushing, subtle vocalizations, and sometimes a glassy-eyed stare. While they can easily be distracted during these masturbatory sessions, attempts to interrupt them are often met with irritability and anger—feelings they will experience again as teenagers when a parent bangs on the bathroom door demanding to know what they are doing in there.

But since adults have blind spots when it comes to childhood sexuality, falsely believing children are devoid of sexual feelings and behaviors until adolescence, when they see their child writhing around making noises like an amorous monkey, it is common for parents to assume their child is experiencing some sort of pain or even a seizure.

This was documented in a series of case studies published in a 2005 article in *Pediatrics* by Dr. Michele Yang and her colleagues. Among the case studies was a two-year-old girl who presented with "spells of back-arching." Beginning a year earlier while sitting in a highchair, the infant would make rhythmic and jerking movements of her arms and legs, accompanied by back-arching and grimacing. The girl remained alert during the episode, but appeared to have a "dazed, distant facial expression."

Her pediatric neurologist conducted EEG and MRI tests, as well as blood screenings for toxin exposure, thyroid dysfunction, and metabolic abnormalities. The infant was prescribed carbamazepine, an anti-epileptic medication. When the neurological and blood tests came back unremarkable, and the medication did not cease the behavior, the physician was left with informing the worried parents that their child is simply a masturbator. Depending on the sexual attitudes of the parents, this conclusion may be worse than a diagnosis of epilepsy.[6]

But unlike epilepsy, infant masturbation does not need treatment. It typically originates through happenstance when the infant explores different parts of their body and realizes that touching their genitals feels good. And similar to many adults, infants are more likely to masturbate when they are tired or stressed. It is a self-soothing behavior like thumb-sucking or body-rocking. Even in cases in which there is high frequency, the occurrence of infant masturbation will generally wane with age due to the child learning a variety of self-soothing behaviors. Therefore, treatment for infant masturbation should be directed at anxious and embarrassed parents who may be tempted to scold or punish their masturbating child. Education may be warranted for parents to better understand how masturbation is normative and healthy, so that parents can learn either to ignore the behavior or to meet their child's stress-reducing needs by offering another interesting, pleasurable, or soothing activity. Although, admittedly, finding a comparable reinforcing behavior to masturbating is a tall order.

Little Sinners

While infant masturbation is well-reported and documented in the scientific literature, self-pleasure more commonly commences during

---

6. Which is why physicians often refrain from saying "infant masturbation" to parents who may think a masturbating infant is a sign of the Antichrist. Instead, physicians often use euphemistic and overly clinical terms like "infantile gratification phenomena," or "infant gratification behavior" to avoid stirring up apocalyptic fears.

prepubescent childhood between the ages of two and twelve. It is during this time that children start becoming curious about the world around them and habitually ask their parents "What's that?" and "Why?" for every unexplained phenomenon. Among them: "Why does Aunt Susan smell like a skunk?" and "What's that buzzing sound coming from your room at night?" Children are attempting to learn about the laws of nature and the norms of society by provoking parents to provide age- and developmentally appropriate answers.

This curiosity is going to naturally extend to one's own body and its functioning. Squeeze your fingertip and it turns purple. Hold your breath and you get dizzy. Laugh too hard and you fart. Touch your genitals and you feel pleasure. But despite the normalcy of childhood curiosity leading to masturbation, it has, historically, been viewed as a sign of child psychopathology.

Dr. Kellogg devoted a significant portion of his 1877 book, *Plain Facts for Old and Young,* to the "foul orgies practiced by the little sinner." He was convinced that the solitary vice caused nail-biting, heart palpitations, enjoying the taste of cinnamon,[7] and "menstrual derangements." Suspicious parents were encouraged to secretly watch their children sleep and abruptly remove their bedsheets and look for signs of penile or clitoral engorgement. If arousal was detected (or if the child attempted to cover their genitals with their hand), then Dr. Kellogg believed the child "may certainly be treated as a masturbator without any error."

To cure children of "defiling themselves," Dr. Kellogg recommended that parents instruct children as early as possible about the physical and spiritual dangers of masturbating. If the scare tactics did not work, bandages over the genitals were suggested. Affixing genital cages or

---

7. If "ketchup is too spicy" was personified, it would look like Dr. Kellogg. He believed the enjoyment of spices was both a cause and consequence of sexual desire and masturbation.

tying the wrists at night were other options, but Dr. Kellogg recognized that determined sinners would often slip out of the restraints or simply turn over and dry-hump the mattress.

But Dr. Kellogg was not the only puritan who tried to prevent a masturbating child from sinking into "driveling idiocy." There were dozens of anti-masturbation devices developed and patented between 1856 and 1918. Dwight Gibbons, for example, patented a spiked metal ring that would stab the child in the penis in the unholy event of getting a nocturnal erection. Although it was not studied at the time, I am guessing there was a high incidence of erectile dysfunction in young adulthood at the turn of the twentieth century.

For psychoanalyst Sigmund Freud, when not obsessing over Oedipal complexes and penis envy, childhood masturbation (either a lack of or "chronic") was a cause of psychopathology, specifically hysteria and neurasthenia (two extremely vague and ill-defined maladies, essentially meaning that "something is wrong with you"). In typical Freudian fashion, he posited overly complex, often untestable theories on the origins and effects of masturbation that are, ironically, just mental masturbation for psychologists.

Even during the second half of the twentieth century and the beginning of the new millennium, childhood masturbation was approached clinically, as opposed to educationally, resulting in harmful punishments administered to children, particularly those with intellectual or developmental disabilities. No longer viewed as a problem in and of itself, clinical intervention during the past sixty years focused on children who masturbated outside the privacy of their bedrooms (e.g., in front of their parents or at school). To treat public masturbation, clinicians in the 1960s used electric shocks and scolding. In the 1970s, clinicians would orally administer lemon juice as an aversion. By the 1990s, physical punishment ceased, but parents were encouraged to take away valued possessions of the "offending" child for transgressions. In the twenty-first century, treatment has focused on eradicating child masturbation with the use of antipsychotic medications.

Even though aversive punishment can be temporarily effective in curbing undesirable behavior under certain conditions, it is an unnecessarily cruel and inhumane way to teach a child about sexual privacy and appropriate places to masturbate. The result of the cruelty, other than the direct implications of inflicting physical harm on a child, is sending the message that masturbation is inherently unhealthy or wrong, resulting in thousands of dollars in sex therapy bills later in life.

What the research on child masturbation informs us, however, is not to approach the behavior punitively, even in cases of inappropriate sexual expression like public masturbation. Given its prevalence, child masturbation is considered normal and developmentally appropriate. This normalcy, however, is dependent on context and the developmental level of the child. For example, according to a paper published in the *European Journal of Pediatrics*, it is common for an infant or a toddler to masturbate in front of others, but it would be uncommon for a twelve-year-old to do so. Children learn social norms and expectations as they age and public masturbation would disappear with this social development, confining self-pleasure to bedrooms, bathrooms, and the occasional kitchen pantry when no one is around. Continued public masturbation for older children would suggest a lack of understanding of society's conventions and would warrant further assessment and treatment from a mental health provider to address why the child is unable to comprehend or conform to social norms. That is not a masturbation problem; that is a developmental problem.

Childhood masturbation with an early onset, typically between the ages of two and five, will wane with age. However, the waning is reflective of parental observations of their child's masturbatory behavior. While it may seem as if the frequency of masturbation is decreasing with age, all that is reported is that the *observation* of the masturbation frequency is decreasing. It is likely the child is simply becoming more secretive when masturbating. Also, there may be an underreporting of girls masturbating compared to boys because of the more covert means of stimulating a clitoris (e.g., subtly rubbing against an object while sitting on the couch) versus stimulating a penis (e.g., hand-stroking the penis in the middle of the living room on Christmas morning).

Other than stimulating the genitals by chance and learning that it feels good, sleep disturbances and breastfeeding weaning can trigger younger children to explore genital stimulation as a way to self-soothe and regulate emotions. Also in younger children, it has been reported that a genitourinary disease like a urinary tract infection can precede the onset of masturbation when the child applies pressure to the genitals in an attempt to ease the pain. When the emotional or physical discomforts subside, the self-stimulation continues for pleasure. For older children, the onset of masturbation may be fostered by social learning through media or friends. Regardless of how they learn about the act of masturbating, children do not have to be taught that it is pleasurable. They do have to be taught, however, to feel ashamed of that pleasure.

Learning Shame

Any time I start a new sexuality class for students or a new sexual health training for therapists, I will ask the audience three questions:

"How many of you grew up in a household where sex was openly discussed? If you had a sex-related question, could you ask one of your parents about it? And would they provide a non-judgmental, medically accurate answer?"

Only a few hands go up, reflecting the rarity of having someone like Dr. Elders as your mother.

"How many of you had the opposite experience growing up? An experience where your parents explicitly said sex was bad, immoral, sinful, or unhealthy (but save it for the one you love). You may have been actively discouraged from even mentioning the topic, even in passing or in innuendo."

A few more hands raise from those who were directly taught shame early on and have spent their adult lives catching up on pop culture that was forbidden to them during childhood like Harry Potter, Tim Burton movies, and the Spice Girls.[8]

"Now how many of you grew up in households someplace in the middle of these extremes? An example of the middle would be that sex just wasn't discussed at all. It wasn't explicitly mentioned that sex should not be talked about in the house, but there was some taboo surrounding it that the topic was simply avoided altogether."

Most of the hands go up.

In so-called "silent families," it is common for parents to completely neglect to talk to their children about sex and masturbation. They are silent because their parents were silent, their parents' parents were silent, and so on up the family tree. It is a family tradition of sexual silence passed down through the generations like a prudish heirloom.

Although there isn't much research on why parents are silent about masturbation, an old study from the 1980s found that parents often have convoluted opinions about their children masturbating. The study found that less than half of parents wanted their sons to have positive

---

8. I crowdsourced these responses from Twitter by asking ex-evangelicals and other former conservative Christians what were some of the pop culture things that were prohibited during their childhood. Other responses included the Smurfs, the Simpsons, Nickelodeon, Pokémon, anything Disney, R.L. Stine books, Care Bears, Barbie dolls, Rugrats, MTV, Troll dolls, He-Man, Cabbage Patch Kids, Rainbow Brite, Barney, and Casper the Friendly Ghost.

attitudes toward masturbation, and only a third of parents wanted the same for their daughters. A quarter of the parents also thought masturbation was harmful to their daughters, but only 9 percent of parents felt similarly about their sons. These negative attitudes (and gender double standards) were related to lower levels of education and higher levels of church attendance among the parents. The more they knelt in church, the more they thought masturbation was self-abuse. But even for the parents who reported permissive or positive attitudes toward their child masturbating, these attitudes were rarely discussed openly with their children.

Given the lack of communication from silent parents about the topic, a study surveying young adults found that they were left to piece together bits of information, myths, and scare tactics to form their own attitudes and perceptions about masturbating while growing up. These attitudes were shaped by religious beliefs, hearing jokes at school about masturbation being "pathetic" because it was a poor substitute for "the real thing," and centuries-old myths about hairy palms and going blind.

Other anecdotal reports talk about the conflicting feelings of these early experiences. On the one hand, masturbation was pleasurable and exciting. On the other hand, masturbation was tainted by feelings of confusion, guilt, and shame afterwards. Not surprisingly, the negative feelings did not last long before the desire to masturbate again returned, only to be replaced by remorse once again. A tortuous shame cycle that can take years (and many therapy hours) to undo.

While threatening hellfire is a surefire way to instill shame and guilt, not discussing masturbation, and actively avoiding it out of discomfort, also send the sex-negative message that masturbation is taboo. It sends the message that masturbation is something different, odd, unique, or "adult" that is not appropriate for children to talk about at the dinner table, let alone engage in under the dinner table when no one is watching.

Innocence or Ignorance?

Even if children are getting shame and guilt instilled into them directly by fear-mongering parents or indirectly by silent parents, an antidote could rest within children receiving comprehensive sexuality education in schools where students simply learn that masturbation is normal. Sex education classes could offer the conversations parents are avoiding and normalize masturbation to reassure millions of anxious children and teens that they will not develop lupus simply by rubbing their genitals for pleasure.

But apparently, that is too much to ask.

It would be nice if we could simply mock the ignorance Dr. Elders experienced in the 1990s as some sort of artifact of a bygone era. Something that did not survive into the new millennium, like Beanie Babies or Vanilla Ice.

But in 2021, history repeated itself. Health and sexuality educator Justine Ang Fonte showed a cartoon video to her first-grade students at a prestigious school in Manhattan's Upper East Side. The video emphasized the importance of knowing our bodies are private. In the video, a cartoon boy stated that he sometimes touches his penis because it feels good. A cartoon girl later chimes in stating that she likes to touch her vulva when she is in the bath or when her mom puts her to bed.

That was it. No real-life depictions of masturbation or genitals. No Disney characters saying that only losers abstain from masturbating. Just a video normalizing touching your own penis or vulva in private.[9]

9. Because the video correctly specified *vulva* instead of *vagina* to refer to the external female genitals, kids who watch it are more knowledgeable about human anatomy than most adults.

Apparently, a few parents (who pay upwards of $55,000 a year to send their seven-year-old to this school) were concerned about their children learning about their own bodies, and they did what the wealthy do best: They complained. The right-wing media ecosystem quickly picked up the story.

Conservative clickbaiter Candace Owens took to Twitter to suggest that Fonte's teaching methods were pedophilic and that she should register as a sex offender. As outlandish as that statement is, it is also an unoriginal and tired trope. It is common for conservatives to label everything that makes them uncomfortable about talking to their kids about sex as "pedophilic" and to call sex educators comfortable enough to do the talking "groomers."

The reality is quite the opposite, ironically. In addition to reducing guilt and shame, masturbation education at an early age is part of sex education aimed at differentiating "good touch" from "bad touch" to increase the likelihood of children reporting sexual abuse. Knowing this difference, as well as having the language to talk about specific sexual body parts, gives children more tools to protect themselves from ongoing sexual abuse and exploitation. Opponents of this education believe they are protecting children from pedophilic sex educators, but the truth is they are making children more vulnerable to sexual predators.

As a sex educator, I've informed many parents that during childhood, "playing with yourself" is just that—play. It is not motivated by sexual desire or aided by sexual fantasies as adolescent and adult masturbation is. And again, this is the challenge for adults to understand and accept. Children have different motivations and mechanisms for masturbating than adults. There is an illogical belief that "allowing" a child to masturbate is inappropriate for the parent. The simple difference between childhood masturbation and child sexual exploitation is to ask who is benefiting from the behavior. If you are simply giving your child privacy to explore their own body because that is what they want to do, that is healthy. If you are initiating the behavior and encouraging it for your own arousal, pleasure, or power, regardless of the child's interest in it, that is abuse.

Simple.

But this Upper East Side school did not understand (or at least did not stand up for) these facts. Bowing to pressure from the same segment of the population who thinks Honduran migrants are going to establish Sharia Law in Arkansas, the school asked for Fonte's resignation. The children of the school are now safe from learning about pleasure, their bodies, and how to recognize abuse.

While right-wing media were upset with the thought of elementary school students being taught the normalcy of masturbation, Fonte's curriculum was in line with the National Sex Education Standards. These standards recommend that by the end of fifth grade, students should understand common occurrences within sexual development, including the onset of masturbation. The World Health Organization's guidelines for sex education also mention that between the ages of five and eight, children should know the parts of their body and their function, and curiosity about these parts and functions is normal. Between the ages of nine and twelve, the guidelines say, students should know that "masturbation does not cause physical or emotional harm but should be done in private."

But this is not happening in public schools in the United States. According to the Guttmacher Institute, thirty-nine states mandate some form of sex education to be provided, but only eighteen states require the education to be medically accurate; only three states prohibit the education from promoting religion; and twenty-eight states require that abstinence be stressed. On top of that, five states require sex education not to "promote homosexuality." And as bleak as all of this is, these are just mandates for the very basics of sex education like contraception and HIV prevention. Masturbation is not a mandated topic to cover in any state, leaving students wondering if what they are doing in the bathroom every day is safe, normal, and healthy.

The closest the United States has come to a mandate for masturbation education in public schools was in California in 2019. The California State Board of Education provided guidelines and tips for K-12 educators who wanted to cover sensitive topics in the classroom. Among them was masturbation, and if it was going to be discussed in the classroom, the manual provided tips for the teachers to cover the topic accurately, such as indicating it does not cause any physical harm. This was not a mandate for teachers to have to teach, but merely some pointers if the topic arose.

Much like the pearl clutching over Dr. Elders twenty-five years earlier, some Californians lost their minds. Protests took place outside the Board of Education in Sacramento the day the guidelines were voted on, with concerned parents holding up signs with an image of the Virgin Mary with the wording "Let children be children." Ironically, given what we know about the frequency and normalcy of childhood masturbation, to "let children be children" would include letting them masturbate.

It should be cautioned, however, that even if the National Sex Education Standards were implemented, there is no guarantee the material would be taught by educators who were competent in objectively leading discussions on childhood and adolescent masturbation. But despite governments restricting what can and cannot be taught about masturbation, global movements of educators and researchers still provide programmatic training to teachers not only to equip them with the skills to address sex-related questions as they arise outside of the curriculum, but also to empirically demonstrate positive outcomes from sex education.

Part of this movement is Dr. Jeno Martin and her research team at Shahid Beheshti University of Medical Sciences in Iran who randomly assigned eighty preschool educators in Tehran to either a sex education training group or a control group. Educators assigned to the training group received sex education within six domains, including masturbation. Educators in the control group received no training. At the end of the two ninety-minute training sessions, educators significantly improved their knowledge of the normalcy of childhood masturbation, as well as significantly decreased punitive attitudes toward a child masturbating. They also demonstrated significantly greater knowledge and more positive attitudes, compared to the control group. Without formal training, educators are at risk of projecting their own biases into the curriculum and perpetuating the myths that abstinence is best and masturbation is a sign of witchcraft.

The push for an abstinence-only approach to sex education is not about sexual health and well-being. It is about religious indoctrination by teaching kids there is only one "right" way to be a sexual being.[10] If abstinence-only education were truly about sexual health, masturbation would be a key topic in its curriculum.

Do you know a sexual behavior that has a zero risk of gonorrhea? Masturbation.

What about a sexual behavior with a zero chance of getting pregnant? Masturbation.

What is a sexual behavior that does not include awkward conversations with a partner about wanting to have intercourse while a Toucan Sam puppet watches?

---

10. "Permissible sex," of course, being sex between a married man and woman, in the missionary position for penile-vaginal intercourse, with the lights off, their eyes closed, and praying for forgiveness afterwards.

Masturbation.

Masturbation teaches pleasure and how the body responds to pleasure. It satisfies sexual drives and desires without the need for a partner. Teaching on the topic ensures that it is normalized as a healthy, developmentally appropriate sexual behavior. But the normalizing of it is condemned by conservatives as harshly as if educators were encouraging raw dogging in the backseat of your mom's minivan behind the local Denny's.

Many parents say that sexuality, including the normalcy of masturbation, should not be taught in schools because those topics are better discussed at home. But we know these conversations are not being held at home. These parents cannot say to schools wanting to offer sex education, "That's my job as a parent" and then get upset when educators teach their kid something the parents have not taught them. That is literally why we pay teachers—to teach kids topics and subjects parents are ill-equipped, reluctant, or do not have the time to teach.

But Representative Dornan's condemnation of Dr. Elders thirty years ago is a reflection of the condemnation of sex education today. The outrage over learning about masturbation, and comprehensive sexuality education in general, is because it challenges "Christian ethics," as Representative Dornan asserted. It challenges the notion that conservative Christianity is a central pillar of sexual health and that its sexual values are universal truths that should be adhered to by all.

Dr. Elders fought back against these clergy crusaders and their apologists, and it is a fight that needs to be waged today to free masturbation from the clutches of ignorance. We are in a unique position to counter masturbation condemnation and the influence of silent families. Whether or not masturbation education exists in our child's school, we can communicate to them that masturbation is a private behavior that is perfectly normal and healthy.

And if you never received any kind of formal masturbation education, let this chapter be your remedial course. Even if you have been a frequent masturbator for the past thirty years, I'm certain you have been bombarded with anti-masturbation messages that may have created some doubt as to whether your history of self-pleasure was healthy or normal. More than likely, the onset, frequency, and manner in which you masturbated during your youth were perfectly normal and healthy, simply because childhood masturbation is normal and healthy. So, take a deep breath and rest assured there was nothing wrong with you, despite what your school principal or pastor may have told you.

CHAPTER 2

Palm Sunday

Priests, Rabbis, and Satanic Masturbation

An orphaned teenager in Uganda, Makko Musagara prayed to God and promised that he would devote his life to Jesus Christ if he could travel far away from his "nagging relatives." When he was offered a scholarship to attend the University of Exeter in England in the mid-1980s, Musagara interpreted this as a miracle and converted to Christianity. Upon returning to Africa after college, he began receiving dreams, visions, and spiritual powers from his new lord and savior where he was able (so he claims) to predict the future, bring children back from the dead, and break the witchcraft curse that was placed on his car's engine that prevented it from operating.

After another series of dreams and visions in 2012, Musagara and his wife felt compelled by God and the Holy Spirit to abandon their business in Kampala and devote their life to building a church and starting a ministry in a remote village over seventy miles north of the Ugandan capital. Musagara's ministry aims to expose "Satan's little-known celestial activities" and protect everyone from the Devil's nefarious goals. One of these "celestial activities" is Satan trying to convince us to masturbate.

In a blog post from 2021 on his website Overcoming Satan, Minister Musagara warns his followers about thirteen reasons masturbation is dangerous to Christians. Along with masturbation being a sin, a possible ticket to Hell, and a detriment to getting and staying married, masturbation "will open a door for Satan and demons to enter your life. Demons of lust, pornography, prostitution, and promiscuity will enter your body and torment you."

On an unexpected side tangent, Minister Musagara also warns that demons have the ability to steal semen after a person masturbates. The demon then takes the semen into the ocean and mixes it with Satan's reproductive fluid.[11] The result of this human-Satan concoction is the creation of mermaids. The minister states, "Masturbating Christians may unknowingly have mermaid offspring in the undersea world."

This is the prequel to *The Little Mermaid* no one asked for.

Admittedly, it is easy to find and mock fringe pastors online spouting nonsense about the mechanisms and effects of masturbation. A simple Google search for "Satan and masturbation" yields a plethora of results that are both entertaining and horrifying, like Christian author (and missed opportunity for a great porn star name) Mack Major who wrote, "Dildos and all of those other sex toys have been used for thousands of years in demonic sex rituals. Masturbation is a direct path to Satan. There's nothing normal about it. And shame on any Christian that says so." Maybe this is just my secular perspective that values a good time, but I don't think talking about demonic dildo rituals is the scare tactic he thinks it is.

It could be argued that it is disingenuous to present these weirdos as representative of the broader religions or religious denominations to which they belong. But aside from mermaids and dildo rituals, their belief that masturbation is fundamentally and unequivocally a sin is deeply rooted in many religions' dogma, particularly Catholicism, Mormonism, Judaism, and Islam.

---

11. It is unclear if Satan ovulates or has some sort of demonic seminal fluid that bonds with human sperm.

For the Bible Tells Me So

Sandwiched in the middle of the Bible's Book of Genesis is the story of
Onan, who was the son of Judah and a nephew of Joseph.[12] After God
killed Onan's older brother for undescribed wickedness, it was com-
manded that Onan marry his brother's widow, Tamar, in order to have
offspring for his dead brother. Not liking the thought of having children
who would not be of his own birthright, when Onan had sex with Tamar
he would withdraw his penis at the timing of orgasm and "spill his seed
upon the ground." God, apparently committed to micromanaging the
behavior of Judah's sons, killed Onan for ejaculating in the wrong place.

The saga continues with twice-widowed Tamar disguising herself as
a sex worker in order to deceive Judah (her father-in-law, mind you) into
having sex in exchange for his seal, cord, staff, and an IOU for a goat.
Months later, gossip spread that Tamar was pregnant from sex work, to
which an enraged Judah called for her to be burned to death immediately. The ever-clever Tamar, however, showed Judah his seal as proof
of his paternity, which spared her life. It's a fable that's fun for the whole
family to enjoy reading at bedtime.

The story of Onan is a cautionary tale of disobedience and the primary biblical justification for prohibiting masturbation. The masturbation term *onanism* derives from this biblical story, as well as the title for
the pseudoscience scare tactic pamphlet *Onania*. However, the sin of
Onan has more to do with not fulfilling a familial duty dictated by God.
It doesn't matter if Onan withdrew his penis at the timing of orgasm
and "spilled his seed" hands-free or if he withdrew his penis and had
to stroke it several times before ejaculating on the ground next to his
sister-in-law. Onan's sin was disobeying God's mandate, not the specific

---

12. Of *Amazing Technicolor Dreamcoat* fame.

mechanism of his disobedience. When sex educators talk about the risks of the withdrawal method, there's warning about the probability of an unplanned pregnancy. But for the believer, the risk of this practice is the probability of being fatally smote by the Almighty.[13]

Beyond the Genesis mandates of obeying God and not wasting seed (which is specific to male masturbation), anti-masturbation religious dogma is also rooted in New Testament passages, primarily Romans 1:24, and 1 Corinthians 6:9 (nice), that indirectly prohibit masturbation for women, too. But much like the story of Onan, these passages do not mention masturbation by name. Instead, the prohibition is against an ambiguous "sexual immorality," which is interpreted to mean any sexual behavior that doesn't exist within a loving marriage for the purpose of procreating the next generation of guilt-ridden Catholic masturbators.

The Pope Is Watching You Masturbate

In 1054, Pope Leo IX wrote a letter, *Ad splendidum nitentis*, condemning masturbation as a gravely disordered act. A position that was reaffirmed by the Catholic church in decrees or declarations under the authority of numerous popes up to and including Pope Benedict XVI in 2012. But it was in 1975 that the church felt compelled to double down on its anti-masturbation stance with the Persona Humana declaration, other-wise known by its more descriptive and less-Latin name: *Declaration of Certain Questions Concerning Sexual Ethics.* In this declaration, the church reaffirms its centuries-old position that masturbation is a grave sin because "the deliberate use of the sexual faculty outside normal con-jugal relations essentially contradicts the finality of the faculty." This

---

13. The withdrawal method is 78 percent effective overall, meaning that Onan still had about a one in five chance of getting Tamar pregnant when he spilled his seed on the ground. Unbe-knownst to him, he had a 100 percent chance of getting executed by God for relying on this unreliable birth control method.

unnecessarily wordy, circularly reasoned justification for prohibiting masturbation is simply saying, "Solo sex is wrong because sex shouldn't be solo."

In summarizing the church's teachings on all things sexual in his 1998 book *Catholic Sexual Ethics*, author and Pittsburgh priest Ronald Lawler warns that our genitals are "not playthings or tools that we are to employ simply for pleasure." Although some argue that one needs to consider contextual nuance, the collared killjoy goes on to state that there are no exceptions to this divine rule. It doesn't matter if you are five years old, or experiencing side effects of a Parkinson's medication that increases sexual desire, or you need to procure a semen sample to test fertility. The act of masturbation, in and of itself, is morally wrong. If infertility testing and treatments weren't stressful enough, now you have the thought of a disapproving priest in the sperm collection room with you.

Despite the strong condemnation of masturbation from the Vatican, unsurprisingly the message is often ignored by the average Catholic. Depending on the study, which varies based on nationality and gender, 60 to 91 percent of Catholics report masturbating, which is not much different from masturbation rates reported by adherents of other religions.

However, Catholics are not a monolith. There are likely significant differences in sexual behavior between members of Cardinals Against Porn and members of Catholics for Choice. One factor that seems to have both a direct and an indirect effect on masturbation frequency is attending Mass. In a 2011 study of Croatian Catholic women, the researchers found an inverse relationship between attending Mass and masturbating, meaning the more someone attended Mass, the less they masturbated. However, a later study in 2018 of French-speaking Catholics (primarily from Belgium) found no relationship between church attendance and rates of masturbation. They did find, though, an indirect relationship. As religious attendance increased, so did sexual guilt, which in turn predicted less masturbation. Whether it's the content of the homilies or the taste of bland communion wafers, there's something about Mass that is related to zapping masturbatory desires.

But still, the majority of Catholics masturbate. There is one subgroup of Catholics, though, known as traditionalists (or Trad Caths in their online spaces), who adhere to the church's strict condemnation of masturbation. They are also traditionalists in every other way within Catholicism and want the church to revert to traditional practices like holding Mass only in Latin and blaming Jews for the world's problems. The fringe of this group, known as radical traditional Catholics (or Rad Trad Caths), have been designated by the Southern Poverty Law Center as a hate group, as they may consist of the largest single entity of anti-semites in the United States.

Unlike mainstream Catholics who may experience passing guilt from masturbating, Trad Caths are gravely concerned with desires to masturbate and will seek counsel from others online to help manage their temptations. One such Trad Cath and self-described "Western Separatist" took to Twitter in 2022 asking for prayers to overcome masturbation addiction. Fellow Trad Caths, or "brothers" as they refer to each other, offered a myriad of ways to reduce or eliminate the temptation to touch your own penis.

The advice included simple competing behaviors that would prevent masturbation or reduce temptations like getting a "dopamine rush" by lifting weights at the gym, deleting Instagram, not spending too much time alone in your room, and, to the delight of the world's owners of capital, getting a second or third job.

Other anti-masturbation suggestions included punitive and restrictive measures to dampen masturbatory urges like taking a cold shower, refraining from consuming meat and dairy, avoiding sugar and caffeine, and fasting completely for forty days. Asked by a brother how fasting was possible for forty days, the Jesus-inspired dietary restrictions were outlined: Only eat less than an equivalent to a small meal per day; no meat on Friday; no eating while the sun is up; no fasting on Sunday; if eating more than allotted occurs, praying for forgiveness commences.

This makes keto seem like a breeze.

Other, more serious Trad Caths offered religious advice not to view masturbation as an addiction but as a sin, something that can be battled with reciting the Apostles' Creed and the Lord's Prayer upon awakening, praying every hour, going to Mass daily to receive the Eucharist, reminding yourself that the Virgin Mary is watching, and keeping a candle lit below your icons at night. However, a priest quickly commented with a warning to make sure the candle is exorcized of demons and blessed before using it.[14]

Viewing masturbation as a sin is aligned with Catholic teachings for the past thousand years, so these Trad Caths are trying to live according to their beliefs. And that should be enough. If you believe masturbation is a sin, then there's no need to conjure up pseudoscientific claims relating to dairy abstinence or doing barbell curls for Christ.

The Catholic theological argument against masturbation is simple: The genitals are made for the sole purpose of expressing love with your spouse and for the possibility of procreation. To deviate from this mandate is to stray from God's plan for your sexuality—a deviation that requires atonement. Within Catholicism, atoning for masturbatory transgressions relies on the individual's ability to take initiative and openly confess their sins to a priest during the sacrament of reconciliation. It's

---

14. Despite my Catholic upbringing, I had to investigate this priest's recommendation. It is a Traditional Roman Rite to exorcize candles in case they have absorbed Satan's power and to bless them, ideally on February 2 during a ceremonial Candlemas—not to be confused with the Swedish doom metal band, Candlemass.

a voluntary admission of guilt, not a coerced confession through inter-rogation. This is in contrast to a long-practiced tradition within the Church of Jesus Christ of Latter-day Saints to investigate masturbation among Mormons.

Masturbating Mormons

Since Mormon teens aren't considered inherently good, to participate fully in Mormon life they must undergo interviews with Mormon elders to determine their worthiness. These interviews are prerequisites for receiving a church calling, going on a mission trip to proselytize to some annoyed stranger, and obtaining a dance card, which is a permission slip to attend a church-run youth dance. I'd imagine those dances are as fun as they sound.

Worthiness, according to the Mormon church, includes chastity for boys and girls who are unmarried. As such, these interviews involve a church elder asking a teen about whether or not they masturbate. The bishop would threaten the child, stating that God would know if they are lying and it would prevent the receiving of blessings. Confessing to sex-ual transgressions, they coercively argue, allows the teen to have a clean slate. It's the Mormon version of a CIA interrogation at Guantanamo.

If the adolescent confesses to masturbating, the minimum punish-ment for the transgression is enduring the shame and awkwardness of being lectured by a seventy-four-year-old man about the dangers of pleasure. More severe punishment could include being denied full par-ticipation in church services, such as taking the sacrament. Imagine the stares and public humiliation as fourteen-year-old Katie stays seated while her family rises to eat some symbolic bread and water—a scarlet M hovering over her head.

The Church of Jesus Christ of Latter-day Saints (LDS) has a long history of participating in moral panic about masturbation. In the late

1800s, church leaders were starting to raise alarms about masturbation affecting young Mormons. Undoubtedly influenced by the circulation of *Onania* and its successors, LDS leadership viewed masturbation as sinful self-pollution that would have dire consequences—spiritual (going to Hell), psychological (going insane), social (unable to get married), and physical (premature death).

In 1958, LDS Apostle Bruce McConkie wrote *Mormon Doctrine*, which explicitly prohibited masturbation, believing that it is a means by which Satan can lead people to Hell. Apostle McConkie was no fan of the secularization of sexuality, particularly after the publication of the Kinsey Reports in the 1940s and 1950s, which revealed that 62 percent of women and 92 percent of men had masturbated at some point in their life. This was a shocking revelation for a culture that assumed only sex offenders and those with mental illness masturbated.[15] McConkie denounced the mental health field's attempts to normalize masturbation in order to alleviate sexual guilt and shame. Guilt and shame, he thought, were symptoms of sin, not symptoms of living within a repressive religion like Mormonism.

In the 1970s, LDS leadership was still pushing back against progress in the medical and behavioral sciences. Mormon elders would warn children that "so-called experts" (i.e., credible psychologists who didn't buy into LDS purity propaganda) may say masturbation is perfectly healthy, but it's important to understand that masturbation shows a lack of self-control that displeases the Lord. As such, masturbation prevention strategies were introduced, like exercising and occupying your hands at night by holding the Book of Mormon and trying to pray

---

15. Dr. Alfred Kinsey, a biology professor from Indiana University, experienced uproar over his publications. Congressman Louis Heller even tried influencing the US Postal Service to block distribution of Kinsey's book on female sexuality, suggesting that its circulation would be "hurling the insult of the century against our mothers, wives, daughters, and sisters."

the urge away. Children and teens were also told that masturbation is not worthy of time and energy because it comes at the expense of noble pursuits like praying and toning Mormon muscles at the gym.

In 1981, an LDS manual for bishops made the lubed-up, slippery-slope argument that masturbation is a gateway to homosexuality by stating, "Early masturbation experiences introduce the individual to sexual thoughts which may become habit-forming and reinforcing to homosexual interests." Although this has been misinterpreted to mean that masturbation can make you gay, the message is that if you are gay, masturbation will fire up your homoerotic interests and make it more likely you'll have sex with someone of the same gender. It is fantasy and thought policing. It is the false belief that as long as you don't think "gay thoughts," you're not gay.

Ultimately, at its core, the LDS masturbation prohibition is similar to the prohibition in Catholicism. Masturbation is a sin simply because it goes against the divine purpose of human sexuality: to express marital love and to make guilt-ridden children.

And much to the dismay of Mormons and Catholics, especially Trad Caths, this is the same rationale used by Jews and Muslims in their condemnation of self-pleasure.

Is Masturbation Kosher and Halal?

Within Judaism, masturbation is condemned, at least indirectly, by rabbinical arguments made in the Talmud, which is a collection of texts that documents centuries of debate among rabbis interpreting Jewish law. The Talmud is like an early version of Reddit that spans hundreds of years. In it, various rabbis interpret and debate the story of Onan and the prohibition of masturbation. The concern is less about masturbation per se, but more about wasteful ejaculation. This is why the rabbis paid little attention to women touching their vulvas because there was no risk of emitting sperm.[16] But because of the possibility of a man ejaculating not for the purposes of procreation, great care had to be taken, for one rabbi warns, "Anyone who emits semen for naught is liable to receive death at the hand of Heaven."

Other rabbis warn that an erection will result in evil inclinations to worship idols, and one was convinced that the wasted seed from masturbation would delay the arrival of the Messiah. Even touching the penis to inspect it for evidence of a nocturnal emission (in which a purification ritual would need to be performed) was frowned upon because touching could lead to arousal and arousal could lead to ejaculation. If one needs to self-inspect, according to an argument in the Talmud, a rock or a piece of earthenware should be used to minimize comfort and pleasure.

One rabbi, Rabbi Eliezer, took this a step further and argued that men shouldn't even touch their penises to urinate. Instead, men should get to an elevated spot and pee hands-free. Other rabbis were concerned that urinating hands-free would result in getting urine on one's garments, which could be a sign that the man doesn't have a penis (logical conclusion, I guess?). This could create public shame if it is believed he could not bear children. Rabbi Eliezer countered these criticisms by saying public shame and embarrassment are better than the moral transgression of holding your own penis to urinate.

Who knew this much impropriety could occur standing at a urinal in a crowded restroom at a Yankees game?

But aside from some communities, these extreme measures are rarely practiced or even considered by most Jews today, with 53 to 100 percent of Jews admitting to masturbating. However, Shmuley Boteach, an American

---

16. They also believed, falsely, that it was not a problem for a woman to touch her vulva to inspect it because women are not capable of sexual arousal from such touching. Patriarchal ignorance about female sexual functioning spared Jewish women from getting direct condemnation.

Orthodox rabbi, has devoted much of his career to the intersection of sexuality and Judaism. In his 2000 book, *Kosher Sex* (as well as subsequent videos on his website), the rabbi argues that masturbation makes spouses less dependent on one another for sexual fulfillment. The goal of sex, he posits, is to act as a joining experience, not an isolating experience. As such, he generally frowns upon it for married people. Rabbi Shmuley is a realist, though, recognizing that single people will masturbate because they lack an available "sexual outlet."[17] However, masturbation among singles is to be viewed as a second-rate behavior, he argues. One should not be satisfied with masturbation as a way to fulfill one's sexual desires. It should be unfulfilling enough to still motivate that person to find their soulmate, suggesting that sexual frustration is a holy motivation to propose marriage.

Within Islam, masturbation is unlawful, as is any sexual behavior outside of heterosexual marriage. Prior to working as a research associate at Memorial Sloan-Kettering Cancer Center, Dr. Sayed Shahabuddin Hoseini published a paper titled "Masturbation: Scientific Evidence and Islam's View" in the *Journal of Religion and Health*. In it, Dr. Hoseini pointed to chapter 23, verses 5–7 in the Quran to justify his interpretation of Islamic law and its prohibition of masturbation: "And they who guard their private parts, except from their wives or those their right hands possess, for indeed, they will not be blamed; but whoever seeks beyond that [in sexual gratification], then those are the transgressors."

Similar to Trad Caths and LDS bishops, Muslim theologians also resort to misleading or outright pseudoscientific claims regarding how masturbation is harmful to one's health. Dr. Hoseini cited several studies

---

17. It has always fascinated me how religious leaders will view masturbation as an objectification of the body, but have no problem viewing one's spouse as a "sexual outlet."

in his article that claimed masturbation is associated with lowered testosterone, increased risk of prostate cancer, and lowered sexual satiation and satisfaction compared to engaging in penile-vaginal intercourse. To avoid masturbating, Dr. Hoseini advised getting married. And if one couldn't marry, then it would be important to fast, take a cold shower, or pray to stave off masturbatory urges. It seems like traditional Catholics and conservative Muslims are strange bedfellows in their strategies to eliminate the sin of touching the genitals.

The dubiousness of the claims made in Dr. Hoseini's paper was confronted by psychology professor David Speed and sociology professor Ryan Cragun. In a published response to the paper in the same journal, Drs. Speed and Cragun point out how Dr. Hoseini presented his argument as a conclusion (masturbation is unhealthy) and cited poorly designed studies to justify his assertion while ignoring scientific evidence to the contrary.

Not surprisingly, this wasn't the first time Dr. Hoseini went out on a pseudoscientific limb about touching your own genitals. In 2007, Dr. Hoseini published an article in *Medical Hypotheses*, titled "Squeezing the Glans Penis: A Possible Maneuver for Improving the Defecation Process and Preventing Constipation." Apparently, according to Dr. Hoseini's two articles focused on touching yourself, there's a fine line between squeezing your penis, which disappoints Allah, and squeezing your penis, which promotes healthy bowel movements.

The empirical data on Muslims and their masturbation habits are similar to those of Catholics and other Christians: As one's Islamic religiosity increases, their masturbation frequency decreases. Additionally, in a study of 297 Muslim university students in Turkey, the greater importance that was placed on Islam (and, in particular, the frequency of attending religious services in a mosque), the more unfavorable attitudes one held regarding masturbation (e.g., it is unhealthy).

So far, religion is painted as not too favorable to masturbating. At its core, the practice is viewed as sinful because it deviates from the divine purpose of sexuality, which is to use one's genitals for the purpose of expressing marital love in hopes of procreation. But the threat of God's wrath from engaging in sin is often not enough to convince people to stop diddling themselves, so theologians, clergypeople, fundamentalists, and even religious scientists have resorted to spouting unverified health effects allegedly stemming from masturbating as a scare tactic to prevent God-fearing people from ending up in a lake of fire. But not all religions share this view of the sacredness of sexuality that has to abide by nonsensical rules.

Hail Satan

In the mid-twentieth century, Anton Szandor LaVey, a local eccentric and nightclub organist, appropriated (but uniquely combined) various philosophical, pagan, and esoteric elements to form a new religious movement. Originally operating solely out of his cottage-style black house in San Francisco, this movement led to the establishment of the Church of Satan on April 30, 1966 (designated as Year One, Anno Satanas). To the horror of parents of baby boomers everywhere, modern Satanism was born.

But much to the disbelief of pastors who feel masturbation is a gateway to the Devil, modern Satanists do not believe in nor worship a literal Satan. Satanism is an atheistic religion, void of any deity supernaturalism. No gods. No masters. Instead, the symbol of Satan has been adopted metaphorically to represent natural human drives and pleasures. Everything the Catholic church has told us to repress, to avoid, or to seek forgiveness and redemption from, Satanism encourages us to embrace.

The seven deadly sins? Guidelines on how to live your best life.

Treat yourself.

Like all religions, Satanism has experienced schisms during its sixty-year history due to disputes over theology and governance, with the formation of The Satanic Temple in the early 2010s (headquartered in the very fitting Salem, Massachusetts), as the most prominent sect apart from the Church of Satan. But despite organizational differences, Satanists are united in their values of individualism, secularism, reason, and pursuits of pleasure.

It is no surprise, then, that Satanism unequivocally endorses masturbation. Published in 1969, LaVey's *The Satanic Bible* devotes an entire chapter to Satanic sex. Within it, LaVey is explicit that all forms of sexual behavior, regardless of how taboo, are permissible if engaged in with consenting partners. LaVey spends considerable time deconstructing the taboos surrounding masturbation, noting that they're the result of religious prohibitions and medical pseudoscience alleging physical, spiritual, and psychological harms.

LaVey also argues that masturbation taboos and restrictions can be destructive to relational and sexual satisfaction. The guilt, secrecy, and insecurities surrounding masturbation can be a harbinger of relational conflict. Additionally, viewing masturbation as a second-tier behavior to "the real thing" will put pressure on couples to have unfulfilling sex together when their sexual needs and satisfaction can often be better achieved alone.

In many ways, Satanism is liberation. To engage in masturbation can be viewed as an expression of one's religious convictions[18] and a way

---

18. Satanism also includes love and lust rituals that incorporate masturbatory orgasms as either a part or the climax of the ritual. For some Satanists, these rituals are performed with supernatural beliefs, similar to magic practiced in other pagan beliefs systems, like Wicca. For others, rituals are performed symbolically. A mechanism of self-focus and empowerment. It's like using a vision board. Only with black candles and vibrators.

to reclaim one's sexuality from the anti-masturbation religious dogma inculcated during their upbringing.

In the 1970 documentary *Satanis: The Devil's Mass*, LaVey discusses the liberating impact Satanism can have on someone's masturbatory guilt and habits. LaVey stated, "Well, I had a man come to me the other day and he said that it was just terrible when he joined the Satanic Church; he was masturbating just about every day. And now he's masturbating two, and sometimes three times a day, and he's very happy. Much happier than he's ever been before."

This anecdote (whether real or mentioned just in jest) of high frequency masturbation is supported by empirical data. My graduate research team at Minnesota State University has investigated Satanic sexuality in a worldwide sample of 908 Satanists. Within that sample, 98.2 percent of Satanists reported masturbating at least occasionally. Just under half (49.1 percent) reported masturbating several times a week or daily. And like the man in LaVey's story, 8.8 percent of Satanists in our study reported masturbating multiple times a day.

It could be argued that Satanism is appealing to those with large sexual appetites for its permissive stance on masturbation; it attracts those leaving a repressive religion and searching for a more accepting, sexually liberated religious home. It could also be argued, however, that these numbers are actually similar to those of other religious groups, but because of the lack of taboo, Satanists are simply more willing to honestly disclose their masturbatory frequencies to sex researchers.

Moderates Masturbating in Moderation

Does this mean that in order for someone to shed masturbation guilt they have to become a Satanist? Although I would personally love to live in a society where the cultural aesthetic looks like a Rob Zombie music video, this is not necessary. There are plenty of avenues to integrate sexuality into religion and spirituality, even biblically. Religious belief can be whatever you want it to be. For every "crucify the flesh" passage, there's a contradictory "his fruit is sweet to my taste" passage.

Sister Margaret Farley, a Catholic nun and professor emeritus of Christian ethics at Yale University, drew the ire and harsh criticism from Pope Benedict XVI in 2012. Her 2006 book, *Just Love: A Framework for Christian Sexual Ethics,* departed from traditional Catholic teachings on masturbation and acknowledged that women "have found great good in self-pleasuring—perhaps especially in the discovery of their own possibilities for pleasure—something many had not experienced or even known about in their ordinary sexual relations with husbands or lovers." She goes on to argue that masturbation may benefit relationships more than hurt them, and, as a result, the decision as to whether or not to self-pleasure is "largely an empirical question, not a moral one." The Vatican was swift in its condemnation, reiterating the buzzkill belief that masturbation is "an intrinsically and gravely disordered action" and warned Catholics not to use the book as a moral guide for sexual expression.

All other religions have their moderates, too. In 2021, Utah-based Mormon and sex therapist Natasha Helfer was excommunicated from the Church of Jesus Christ of Latter-day Saints because she spoke out against the church's policies regarding sexuality, including masturbation and pornography.

Dr. Ruth Westheimer, a Jewish woman who escaped Nazi persecution during her childhood in Europe, went on to become one of the world's leaders in sex therapy and education in the 1980s, often promoting the benefits of masturbation.

Dr. Tariq Al Habib, a Saudi Muslim psychologist, argued on television in 2018 that masturbation is a human need and that Islamic scholars need to reevaluate their condemnation of it. Earlier that year, Saudi Muslim youth trended the hashtag #MasturbationIsHalal on Twitter, arguing that solo sex is (or at least should be) permissible within Islam.[19]

Granted, taking a straightforward, centuries-old condemnation of masturbation requires some mental gymnastics and a certain degree of secularization to reinterpret it progressively. But it's the same process that has eased the rigidity for dietary restrictions, using birth control, interfaith marriages, and the use of technology. Pastors, priests, rabbis, and imams of yore would be outraged by the lifestyle of even the most conservative and traditional religious adherents today. The wealth and idolatry in modern culture alone would undoubtedly have Jesus flipping tables at a hipster farmer's market in Brooklyn that sells "Coexist" bumper stickers.

The dominant world religions prohibit masturbation because of the belief that the genitals are supposed to be used only for one function. But why can't there be more than one function? Even if we suspend reason, dismiss everything we know about how humans have evolved, and believe that God designed us, it's not a huge leap to argue that our body parts can have several, God-given roles.

The spine and its connective tissue, for example, can be viewed as specifically designed to allow us to walk and sit upright, freeing our hands to multitask and giving us an edge over many other species on this planet. We can walk while pushing shopping carts, and we are able to grab a box of Pop-Tarts from the top shelf to ensure our survival. So even if the primary function of our spine and back is to allow bipedalism, don't these body parts also allow us to experience pleasure? Can we

---

19. However, Saudi high school teacher Muhammad al-Sahimi was sentenced to three years in prison and three hundred lashes for saying something similar during a lecture on love in Arabic poetry. A reminder that if you're going to challenge religious teachings where it is illegal to do so, have privacy, security, and legal protections in place.

not enjoy soaking our back in a bath or sitting in a massage chair while a vibrator pounds our lumbar? Our genitals can be viewed as having multiple purposes as well.

As an atheist, I find it hard to imagine worshipping a god who, despite creating 100 billion galaxies in the observable universe, is really mad about your dildos. I'd argue that there's no reason to worship gods or to fear monsters. But if theistic belief is important to you, at least worship a god who is cool with you masturbating in the shower.

The god assigned to you at birth does not have to be yours for your entire life. If it is religion and spirituality you seek, find a religious and spiritual home that aligns with your pleasure. Do not torture yourself trying to adhere to sexual rules you don't agree with. Dismiss the hellfire scare tactics that you don't even believe in. If you think Hell is fake, feel free to masturbate.

Once the spiritual battle is won and you no longer believe Satan is using masturbation to send you to Hell, the battle toward liberation continues against health hucksters and insecure men trying to convince you that ejaculating will cause disease, disability, and death.

CHAPTER 3

Semen, the Magical Elixir

Retention, Culture-Bound Syndromes, and Insecure Incels

A twenty-two-year-old man from Mumbai, India, recently underwent reconstructive surgery at a urology clinic located in a northeastern suburb of the city. Three years earlier, he was very distressed over fears he was losing semen every time he urinated. He worried that this semen loss would eventually result in physical weakness, erectile dysfunction, and a host of severe diseases. Finding no anxiety relief, even after numerous visits to traditional healers and physicians, he took matters into his own hands and cut off his penis.

The now-penis-less man suffered from *Dhat syndrome*, a condition marked by an intense fear of losing semen, and accompanied by symptoms of fatigue, weakness, sexual dysfunction, and depression. Given the Hindu medical belief in seven essential bodily fluids—semen being one of them—concern about losing this essential fluid is widespread in India and Pakistan. Among men seeking psychiatric care in India for sexual complaints, 64 percent of the patients experience Dhat syndrome, whereas 30 percent of men seeking general medical care in Pakistan also report symptoms consistent with Dhat.

In the *Diagnostic and Statistical Manual of Mental Disorders* (DSM-5), Dhat syndrome is only listed as a "culture-bound syndrome," which is a cluster of symptoms that exists as a phenomenon only within specific cultures. *Koro* is another example of a culture-bound syndrome, which is found primarily in Southeast Asia and is marked by the delusional belief that one's penis is shrinking and will eventually disappear.[20]

With Dhat being labeled only as a culture-bound syndrome, the American Psychiatric Association is suggesting that fear of semen loss is unique to only a few foreign cultures and shouldn't be found among white Instagram wellness influencers from Seattle.

But this is not the case.

Fearing the effects of losing semen through voluntary or involuntary means is not tied to a specific culture, but tied to a more general belief that ejaculating from masturbation is physically unhealthy. This has existed in American and European culture for centuries, and explains why everyone from nineteenth-century temperance proponents to twenty-first-century wellness grifters believe that the key to health is preventing semen from leaving your body.

Sexy S'mores

Several decades before Dr. Kellogg's anti-masturbation toasted corn flakes hit the shelves, Sylvester Graham, an evangelical minister from Connecticut, was concerned with the moral decay of nineteenth-century America. Although he was a minister who often spoke about sin and hellfire, Reverend Graham relied on an amateur's understanding of physiology and used medical jargon to masquerade as an expert in the medical sciences. His reactionary sexual beliefs, more so than any

---

20. Not all culture-bound syndromes involve the genitals or sexual functioning. *Hwa-byung*, for example, is a culture-bound syndrome found among Korean women. The syndrome involves the woman feeling as if she has an abdominal mass (despite none being physically detected on physical examination), and the syndrome is believed to be caused by a suppression of depression or anger. This is a common theme among many culture-bound syndromes, where physical complaints stem from psychological distress, supporting the importance of feeling your feelings and occasionally crying in the shower listening to Taylor Swift.

formal medical knowledge, influenced his assertion that masturbation would "inflame the brain more than natural arousal" and result in debilitating illness.

In 1837, he published *A Lecture to Young Men on Chastity* to scare boys, the parents of boys, and young men into sexual temperance and masturbation abstinence. The list of ailments he believed was caused by this unnatural vice is immense and included violent belching, diarrhea and other "discharges from the anus," bleeding from the mouth and nostrils, feeling as if ants were crawling under the skin, a chilling sensation in the spine, a cadaver-like appearance, tooth loss, cerebral hemorrhage, spontaneous abortion, bloody semen, burning penis, and suicide.

If this list of symptoms and diseases didn't paint a clear picture of what a self-polluter looks like, Reverend Graham summed it up in vivid detail:

... the wretched transgressor sinks into a miserable fatuity, and finally becomes a confirmed and degraded idiot, whose deeply sunken and vacant, glossy eye, and livid, shriveled countenance, and ulcerous, toothless gums, and fetid breath, and feeble, broken voice, and emaciated and dwarfish and crooked body, and almost hairless head—covered, perhaps, with suppurating blisters and running sores—denote a premature old age—a blighted body—and a ruined soul!—and he drags out the remnant of his loathsome existence, in exclusive devotion to his horridly abominable sensuality.

One must wonder how vigorously Reverend Graham believed people masturbated.

Although there is passing mention in Graham's text about harm to women's bodies when experiencing sexual arousal and orgasm, there is a reason this book was written specifically for boys. The reverend saw the modernization of New England Yankee culture as a deviation from the hierarchical and patriarchal New England Puritan culture that preceded it. Masturbation amounts to a crisis of masculinity. To become a man, a male must only act on his sexual motivation by engaging in sexual intercourse with a woman. To do otherwise, men are violating masculine scripts and demonstrating a weakness of character, unable to control their sexual urges. Furthermore, the physical result of this lack of self-control is the list of Graham's WebMD ailments, which leads to a weakening (i.e., feminizing) of the male body.

To prevent the decay of wretched transgressors, Reverend Graham promoted a diet primarily consisting of vegetables, water, and whole grains. Shying away from modernization and the use of refined flour, the reverend advocated for only using whole wheat flour that would not only prevent a "lazy colon" but also the sins of the flesh. This flour served as the foundation for a bread, ultimately becoming known among his faithful followers as "graham crackers."

Much like corn flakes, the belief that graham crackers have any influence on someone's sexual desire and masturbatory urges is solely based on moralistic pseudoscience. Crackers, whether manufactured by Nabisco or promoted by a religious zealot, will not prevent you from wanting to touch your genitals. The next time you're gathered around the campfire, feel free to enjoy a solo orgasm with your s'mores.

But almost two hundred years later, these distorted beliefs about masturbation (rooted in moral objection, pseudoscience, and reactionary politics) persist with similar fervor. Masturbatory abstinence is still viewed as the solution to the problem of bodies not achieving a masculine ideal and is promoted by angry internet bros disguised as spiritual wellness coaches.

Easy Cum, Easy Go: Semen Retention

In 2022, I created a series of posts on Instagram debunking some basic assertions about the physical benefits of masturbation abstinence. It didn't take long before self-described healers and wellness coaches stopped by my comments to call me ignorant and an imperialist for thinking that Western science can falsify claims made by ancient Eastern philosophies. Not surprisingly, these healers and wellness coaches were mainly white guys from Portland with tribal tattoos.

With the smell of patchouli in their dreads, these guys have adopted Chinese, Tibetan, and Indian philosophies into their own influencer brand, and felt as if I was, in their words, "shitting on" their ancient beliefs. They claim to be practitioners, or at least believers, of Taoism and Traditional Chinese Medicine, and seem to have an unhealthy fixation on the Taoist beliefs relating to semen retention.

Within Taoism, *qi* is the overall life force and *jing* is often associated with semen, another important source of energy. According to this belief, when semen is ejaculated, a person's jing decreases, which in turn diminishes their qi. When both are depleted, the person dies.[21]

Therefore, the goal of semen retention is to maintain jing in order to bolster qi. But this doesn't necessarily mean a life of celibacy. The person is still able to have sex, but instead of ejaculating, they internalize that seminal energy and apply it to other parts of their body in a process known as "sexual transmutation." I did a scholarly article search to learn more about the scientific processes of sexual transmutation, but only found papers like "From Teosinte to Maize: The

---

21. For some Taoists, you may already be screaming this is a misunderstanding of jing. Maybe so, but I'm not alone. Zhang and Rose (1999) identified twenty-two different definitions of jing. Much like all religions and spiritualities, it's make it up as you go along.

Catastrophic Sexual Transmutation," which is about the reproductive evolution of corn.

Much like the dominant religions discussed in the last chapter and their view of masturbation being a sin, I could accept (albeit disagree with) a Taoist spiritual or metaphysical assertion that semen has immeasurable energy that is depleted during ejaculation. But once that spiritual belief is elaborated on with pseudoscientific biochemical processes, then those beliefs can be "shit on."

In his seminal book *The Tao of Sexology*, author and founder of the Foundation of Tao Dr. Stephen Chang attempts to quantify this ejaculatory energy loss. He states that in every tablespoon of semen there is nutritional value that "is equal to that of two pieces of New York steak, ten eggs, six oranges, and two lemons combined." If true, we should be concerned about the cholesterol risks of giving a blow job.

According to Dr. Chang, the exhaustion a man feels after ejaculation is due to semen's "vital energy" escaping the body. Instead of the slang term *coming*, he prefers ejaculation be called *going* because "everything—the erection, vital energy, millions of live sperms, hormones, nutrients, even a little of the man's personality—goes away. It is a great sacrifice for the man, spiritually, mentally, and physically."

To prevent the travesty of semen loss, but to retain an active and pleasurable sex life, Dr. Chang recommends pressing on your perineum (or the "Million Dollar Point" as he grossly calls it) during orgasm. By doing so, he believes this will prevent the immediate and fast expulsion of semen, and instead will allow the prostate to slowly spew the fluid into your bloodstream. This allows the body to retain the vital nutrients and energy in semen. The mechanism of this process is not fully explained in the text, but it somehow involves "lubricating and coating the nerves" in a way that will prevent multiple sclerosis.

In Daniel Reid's *The Tao of Sex, Health, and Longevity*, the horrors of semen loss are "written from a Westerner for the Western mind." Reid argues that semen is more difficult on your body to replenish than blood, and that ejaculating more than twice a month leads to chronic fatigue, low energy, irritability, and a loss of interest in your partner. Out of nowhere, Reid asserts that 20 percent of semen is made up of cerebrospinal fluid and, as a result, could lead a daily masturbator to psychosis.

Since the focus of concern is on semen and ejaculation, women are typically neglected in conversations about the supposed benefits of masturbation abstinence. Reid only mentions women in passing, suggesting that they are not impacted by the deleterious effects of an orgasm because, according to him, women have an "inexhaustible" sexual appetite.

Also of concern is the amount of zinc in semen. According to this pseudoscientific belief system, when this zinc-rich semen is ejaculated, it leads to memory loss and hypersensitivity to sunlight. Essentially, I guess, turning someone into a vampire with Alzheimer's.

Both Reid and Dr. Chang are concerned about the vital nutrients in semen that your body supposedly depends on for wellness and even survival. If you're convinced that such nutrients exist and are lost during ejaculation, couldn't you just eat your semen after ejaculation like a multivitamin?

Strangely, this advice was not mentioned in either text.

Admittedly, I didn't know anything about Taoism prior to writing this chapter. But I didn't have to. I know ejaculating is not harmful to your body and retaining semen is not doing your body any favors. It would be akin to the latest Spider-Man movie claiming that Peter Parker could ejaculate out of his wrists. I wouldn't have to know anything about the Marvel Cinematic Universe in order to confidently dismiss that claim as fiction.[22]

Which brings us back to the overly confident white wellness gurus on Instagram. When I made a post dismissing the false belief of semen's magical powers and that you can enjoy a worry-free orgasm, a fire dancer and somatic movement practitioner named Tomcat was quick to argue that just because the life force energy isn't measurable, that doesn't mean men aren't drained of energy after ejaculating. Feeling masochistic, I responded, seeking to understand what Tomcat believes to be the underlying physical processes of energy as they relate to semen loss.

Tomcat focused his argument on the belief that, during ejaculation, there is a burst of energy expenditure and a loss of glucose from the muscles. He feels that by not ejaculating, the body is storing this energy and that it can be expended during more important psychological tasks. He also argued that by abstaining from ejaculating, your body learns to save this energy and compound it over the person's life. To which my first thought was a seventy-five-year-old whose body is made up of 90 percent stored cum energy.

Giving him room to dig a deeper intellectual black hole, I asked him if what he's describing has more to do with orgasm than semen loss, and what kind of impact this has on those without prostates and seminal vesicles. Tomcat, enthusiastic to share his wisdom, quickly responded by saying that ejaculation requires more energy than orgasm, and that women can also experience this to a degree, but since they have less muscle mass, they're not impacted by it too much. And for those who have had their prostates and seminal vesicles removed because of cancer

---

22. I'm assuming someone already wrote this as fan fiction and is waiting for Disney to option the script.

and therefore can no longer ejaculate, Tomcat believes they benefit from having semen stored in their bodies without a means of escaping.

At that point, I realized I was conversing with an idiot.

Not an idiot for simply being ignorant about the complexities of semen, orgasm, and ejaculation, but an idiot because he thought he was an expert on the complexities of semen, orgasm, and ejaculation. What it must be like to walk through the world with so little knowledge, but so much confidence.

Sadly, culturally appropriative Taoists aren't the only insufferable semen retentionists who exist on social media. There are other groups of men who have found online solidarity in their shared passion for idealized masculinity, hating women, and not coming.

A Month of Nonsense: No Nut November

Immediately following the indulgence and revelry of Halloween on October 31, No Nut November begins to trend across social media platforms. Not to be confused with a campaign promoting anti-cashew bigotry, No Nut November is a challenge to abstain from masturbating (i.e., "nutting") for the month of November.

It's an extension of the other challenge during the month of November, called Movember, where men attempt to grow mustaches for thirty days to raise awareness about men's health issues like prostate cancer. It is ironic these two challenges occur in the same month because there is an association between *higher* frequency of ejaculation and *lower* risk of prostate cancer (involving almost 32,000 men in a twenty-year study measuring ejaculation frequency from both partnered and solo sex). Research that looks at the association of ejaculation only from masturbation and prostate cancer risk is less common, but one analysis of sixteen existing studies did suggest a correlation. Half of those studies analyzed suggested that more masturbation could mean less prostate cancer risk. The other half of the studies found no relationship.

For most participants of No Nut November, however, the challenge is a harmless joke where people race to post a meme at 12:01 a.m. on November 1, indicating how they already failed the challenge. For others, it is reminiscent of the classic *Seinfeld* episode, "The Contest," where George vows never to masturbate again after his mother catches him "treating his body like an amusement park," which prompts him, Jerry, Elaine, and Kramer to place bets to see who can abstain the longest. Among close friends, it's an opportunity to engage in low-stakes competition, trying to tempt each other by texting porn gifs and links to their favorite celebrity sex video.

But as journalists Samantha Cole and Ej Dickson have reported, No Nut November has a deeper meaning among those who find no joy in a viral hashtag. For these downers, No Nut November is a solemn reminder of their vows of masturbatory chastity in their quest to become the manliest of men.

Part of the "manosphere" (which includes men's rights activists, pickup artists, and incels),[23] these guys have taken to message boards, YouTube, and most recently TikTok to complain about the feminization of society and to share their strategies for upping their manliness. Regularly calling people cucks, betas, soy boys, and (my personal favorite) soft cunts for not living up to a hypermasculine ideal, these weirdos have

---

23. Involuntary celibates, self-described as "incels," are men who are very upset over the fact they do not have a girlfriend. They want to be having sex, but no one wants to have sex with them, hence the involuntary nature of their celibacy. Instead of recognizing that most people aren't able to have sex every time they want to and are therefore, by definition, incels as well, these guys adopt the label as a significant identity. What separates the incel from everyone else not having sex is a grandiose sense of entitlement that they *should* be having sex, and it is the world's worst injustice that they are not.

become fixated on their own physical and sexual insecurities and have devoted their lives to trying to achieve and maintain "alpha" status.

Of primary concern is testosterone and how they believe masturbation decreases this sex hormone. This, they believe, prevents them from chiseled jawlines and, ironically, "cum gutter" abs.[24] Through masturbation abstinence, they feel they can boost their testosterone and end up looking like a Spartan from *300*. Once they achieve this ideal masculinized physique, they will no longer be single because now they have something to offer women to compensate for their annoying personality, antiquated gender scripts, and scientific illiteracy.

However, their assertion that masturbation decreases testosterone is not conclusively supported by research. The most common study abstainers offer as evidence is a 2003 study from China that found increased levels of testosterone after seven days of abstinence. The study, measured from twenty-eight participants, mind you, found similar company in a 2001 German study that only involved ten participants and found higher testosterone levels among men after a period of three weeks of abstinence. It should be noted that the widely cited 2003 study was retracted by the journal in 2021 after it was discovered the article had already been published in Chinese in another journal, two out of the four researchers could no longer be found, and the remaining researchers refused to provide the raw data for review by those unaffiliated with the original study. Therefore, the entire argument that masturbation decreases testosterone is based on the hormone levels of ten temporarily abstinent Germans from over twenty years ago.

Even if this were compelling evidence, it is in contrast to studies that have found relationships between high masturbation frequency and

---

24. In case you wanted to impress your coworkers with the latest sexual slang, "cum gutter" abs refer to well-defined, V-line abdominal muscles that would act as a viaduct for semen when ejaculated onto.

high testosterone, as well as increases in testosterone after masturbating to porn and watching people have sex at a swingers' club.

All of these studies suffer from methodological limitations, particularly small sample sizes. Sadly, it's difficult to recruit thousands of people willing to masturbate (or abstain from masturbating) for science, and even more difficult to convince the federal government to fund the research. As a result, the body of literature on the relationship between masturbation and testosterone is inconclusive. It is a misrepresentation of the data to assert that masturbation abstinence will significantly increase your testosterone, just as it would be a misrepresentation of the data to assert that masturbating to an OnlyFans video will significantly increase your testosterone.

In response to one of my many innocuous "masturbation is healthy" posts on Instagram, one of these young men thought I was being irresponsible and reckless in my normalization of self-pleasure. He felt compelled to share his experience of feeling depressed, having low self-esteem, lacking motivation, and difficulties lifting weights at the gym whenever he masturbates.

I became inquisitive and wanted to learn more about this somatic experience. He believed that frequent ejaculation kills his masculinity, and that, by abstaining, he is able to experience boosts in his testosterone that allow him to have deeper squats and more confidence to approach an uninterested woman to ask her about her tattoos.

Curious about his perception of this experience, I asked if he is distressed that an orgasm causes him to feel this way, especially considering that is not a common response for most people who masturbate. He quickly became defensive and said that there is nothing wrong with him. He just needs to work a little harder if he "relapses."

It's a pull-yourself-up-by-your-own-chastity-belt mindset of self-empowerment.

What compounds this fear is misinterpreting normal bodily sensations after orgasm as a sign of disease. When orgasm is near, dopamine spikes, but the neurotransmitter is quickly inhibited by increases in prolactin,[25] oxytocin, endocannabinoids, and endorphins after orgasm. For most people, this neurochemical experience results in feelings of relaxation, contentment, and ease. It's why many people will masturbate before bed to help them sleep. But for the anxious masturbator, these feelings of relaxation are misinterpreted as feelings of fatigue and weakness and will have them convinced every ejaculation is depleting them of their masculine energy.

Admittedly, the abstinence advocates are partially correct in their knowledge: Semen does contain energy and vital nutrients. The misunderstanding is who or what benefits from the energy and vital nutrients. The reality is that only the sperm cells benefit, not the person making the sperm cells. Either by giving the cells energy or by making their journey more hospitable, semen only exists to increase the survival of sperm.

Your body does not rely on, nor benefit from, the biochemical components of semen. The un-ejaculated semen that would slowly get absorbed into the person's body has such a trace amount of nutrients that your body treats it as a triviality.

For example, Daniel Reid and his Taoist disciples believe the loss of zinc during ejaculation leads to memory loss and hypersensitivity to sunlight. While zinc is an important mineral for our bodies (primarily for cell growth for immunity and healing), the average amount of zinc

---

25. Prolactin is a hormone secreted by the pituitary gland and is responsible for mammary gland development and milk production for women who are pregnant or breastfeeding. For those not pregnant or breastfeeding, prolactin exists in low amounts. However, this can ignorantly be interpreted by semen retentionists as evidence of the "feminizing" effects of masturbation. But the prolactin increase post-orgasm is slight and brief, and it simply results in temporary feelings of sexual satisfaction and satiation. Rest assured, nervous abstainers, no amount of ejaculating will ever result in growing breasts and lactating.

that is in semen is 0.561 mg. For reference, adult men are recommended to consume 11 mg of zinc per day. Even if the body were dependent on its zinc intake from reabsorbed prostate fluid (it isn't), that would only be 5.1 percent of the daily recommended amount. This is equivalent to eating only six cashews, which makes No Nut November even more ironic.

A Community of Wankers Not Wanking: NoFap

In 2021, Marlene Hartmann, a sociology research fellow at the University of Technology in Chemnitz, Germany, published an article in *Sexualities,* critically examining the content of the eleven most-watched videos on YouTube that preach the gospel of NoFap. Started in 2011, NoFap began as a subreddit where guys could support one another in abstaining from masturbation, particularly masturbation while watching pornography. While there is conflation between masturbation, pornography, and orgasm within this community, and which one is the greatest of the three evils, Hartmann's analysis focused more on the themes specifically within the discourse of masturbatory orgasm abstinence.

Similar to Reverend Graham's concerns, men spouting off on YouTube about the benefits of masturbation abstinence had a masculine ideal that included a natural body (a strong desire to have sex with women) and a cultured mind (the ability to master one's desires). Masturbation deviates from this ideal by focusing sexual energy on the self and not being manly enough to resist the urge to do so.

According to one video, masturbatory orgasm "is a reward that is normally only achievable by meeting a potential mate, coming off as an attractive mate, and eventually growing the balls to make a move and having sex." The commentator makes an assumption about sexual normalcy, suggesting that effort is needed to obtain the reward of orgasm. Masturbation circumvents this "natural" order by reducing the amount of effort men need to exert in order to experience sexual pleasure—pleasure that should only come from sex with women after having earned it through hard work.

Masturbatory desire, as opposed to the so-called natural desire to put a penis into a vagina, is viewed as effeminate. In order to overcome these urges, one simply needs to man up, as one video creator eloquently stated: "The biggest thing that I realized is that if you wanna get over this, you gotta stop being a little bitch."

If only behavioral modification were this easy, psychologists would have the luxury of simply calling their patients "little bitches" and seeing remarkable therapeutic progress.

But it was the armchair evolutionary psychologist YouTuber who laid out what is happening when you finally start abstaining from masturbating: ". . . your brain starts to provide you with the tools to have the highest chance possible to start attracting the opposite sex to reproduce. This is where the 'super-powers' come in: the confidence, the motivation, the drive to make money, the burning desire to leave your mark on this world. All of these benefits stem from your brain giving you the highest chance to reproduce."

The fixation of NoFap on reproduction is interesting because it is true that abstinence leads to higher volume of seminal fluid and a higher number of sperm cells (because they're being "stockpiled" by not being ejaculated). However, abstinence does not make the sperm healthier in terms of better motility, morphology, or vitality. Further, this abstinence effect plateaus after a couple of days, meaning a weekly masturbator and an abstainer have equal chance that intercourse with a woman will result in pregnancy. What's also important to note is that any abstinence effect is caused by total abstinence, not just abstaining from masturbation. Your testes and sperm cells do not care if you're ejaculating onto your iPad or having Vatican-approved sex on your honeymoon.

And the rest of your body doesn't care, either. An orgasm is an orgasm. NoFappers, retentionists, or other abstainers who report feeling depressed, weak, and guilty after masturbating are not feeling that way because their body is punishing them for "wasting their seed." They feel that way because of their distorted beliefs about masturbation.

Dr. Nicole Prause, a neuroscientist at the University of California, Los Angeles, studied NoFappers and their attempts to abstain from masturbating. In addition to a high level of narcissism among the study's participants, she found that abstainers who recently "relapsed" reported feeling ashamed, worthless, and suicidal. These feelings were fueled by engaging in online NoFap or "reboot" forums where 23.5 percent of these tormented masturbators reported seeing encouragement to harm or kill themself.

This is why treating a fear of ejaculation often needs clinical intervention, not self-help or peer support from NoFappers. Of the few studies that have focused on this treatment, it was found that symptoms were alleviated by antidepressant medications, therapy focused on irrational fears, and sex education about the normalcy of masturbation and ejaculation. Unsurprisingly, validating the fear of ejaculating and encouraging masturbation abstinence have never been demonstrated to give anxious people masculine superpowers.

Ejaculation 101

A lot of the misinformation about semen wouldn't exist if we had received comprehensive sex education instead of just being shown vintage pictures of untreated herpes from the 1960s. So, let's review the basics.

Semen is the broad term for all of the fluid, ions, sugars, proteins, and germ cells that are ejaculated during orgasm. The word *semen* is often used interchangeably with the word *sperm*, but sperm cells (developed in each testicle and stored in each epididymis) make up only between 1 percent and 5 percent of the total volume of semen. And while the evolutionary purpose of ejaculation is to release those sperm cells, the rest of the seminal fluid is there to aid, nourish, and protect those cells. Think of semen as the Vatican Swiss Guard for sperm.

In addition to the sperm cells, 5 percent of semen's fluid volume comes from the Cowper's gland, 15 to 30 percent from the prostate gland, and the majority comes from the seminal vesicles. The Cowper's gland fluid is an alkaline mucus consisting of glycoproteins produced during sexual arousal that neutralizes the acidity of the urethra to allow safe passage for the sperm. The prostate secretes a milky-colored fluid during ejaculation and contains acid phosphatase, citric acid, inositol, zinc, calcium, and magnesium to support the mobility of the sperm cells. The seminal vesicles add fructose, ascorbic acid, and prostaglandins to the ejaculatory cocktail, giving sperm cells more energy for their squiggly voyage.

During orgasm, smooth muscle contractions of the epididymis, vas deferens, prostate, and seminal vesicles combine with sphincter contractions of the same genitourinary tract. This coordinated dance of contractions, along with each gland and vesicle's unique biochemical fluid, serves the interests of the sperm cells on their journey to the fallopian tube or shower drain.

CHAPTER 4

Addicted to Self–Diagnosing

Masturbation Addiction, Moral Incongruence, and Expensive 12 Steps

I n November of 2009, music cable channel VH1 debuted *Sex Rehab with Dr. Drew.* Coming off the successful heels of Dr. Drew Pinsky's *Celebrity Rehab,* the new show documented a twenty-one-day residential treatment program for actors, models, musicians, and pro athletes battling some form of sex addiction and waning celebrity status.

Taking place at the Pasadena Recovery Center, Dr. Drew opened each episode with voice-over narration saying that sex addiction is just as deadly as alcohol and drug addiction. Failing to elaborate on how someone can fatally overdose from vibrators just as easily as from fentanyl, Dr. Drew introduced the patients (i.e., cast members) who have agreed to enter treatment under the strict rules of no touching, no "inappropriate dress," no pornography, and no masturbation for three weeks. It was like a monastery for D-list celebrities.

Porn star Penny Flame (who later admitted to joining the show to boost her career) was the first to stir drama and violate the rules by smuggling a sex toy in her luggage, which the treatment staff considered contraband and quickly confiscated like it was a crack pipe. Each episode had the standard and essential elements of a popular reality TV program—dramatic music, rehearsed verbal arguments, physical assaults, and tears.

So many tears.

Sex Rehab was like most cable reality TV shows in the early 2000s, and is easily forgettable. What shouldn't be forgotten, however, is Dr. Drew's role in perpetuating our culture's ignorance and fear about masturbation by mischaracterizing and sensationalizing "sex addiction" to boost his own Hollywood stardom.

Dr. Drew is a board-certified physician and addiction medicine specialist in the state of California, and of note is his double role as the attending physician and the executive producer for *Sex Rehab*. This dual relationship with the patients has been a source of controversy within the addiction field, as the director of the Substance Treatment and Research Service at Columbia University, Dr. John Mariani, told the *New York Times Magazine*: "The problem here is that Dr. Drew benefits from [the patients'] participation, which must have some powerful effects on his way of relating to them. He also has a vested interest in the outcome of their treatment being interesting to viewers, which is also not in their best interest. Treatment with conflicts of interest isn't treatment." In other words, if you're serious about seeking treatment for a sexual disorder, make sure your doctor's clinic isn't listed on IMDb.

It was inevitable that the sensationalism behind "masturbation addiction" was going to become reality TV entertainment. Pathologizing normal sexual behavior makes compelling television viewing, and an easy way to secure a large audience and generate revenue from thirty-second ads for Nutri-Grain bars. And while Dr. Drew capitalized on this for television fame, he wasn't the first and isn't the only physician or therapist to believe excessive masturbation is just as deadly as drug addiction and to advocate for using untested cures for anxious masturbators.

The Birth of a New Disease

After signing the Declaration of Independence and serving as the surgeon general in the Continental Army during the Revolutionary War,

Dr. Benjamin Rush became gravely concerned about the sexual well-being of Americans. In his 1812 book *Medical Inquiries and Observations Upon the Diseases of the Mind*, Dr. Rush devotes an entire chapter to "The Morbid State of the Sexual Appetite," expressing concern with an over-interest in sex, especially in the form of masturbation.

Dr. Rush presented a number of cures for excessive masturbation, which seem to be a hodgepodge of anecdotes and assumptions about what can decrease masturbatory desires. He recommended long journeys on horseback, getting married, bathing in cold water, avoiding obscene conversations, listening to certain tones of music, engaging in a sudden fit of laughter, studying mathematics,[26] taking laxatives, waging war to achieve military glory, and not looking at a woman directly in the face. According to Dr. Rush, women responding to a cleavage-gazing man with "eyes up here" would only heighten his arousal.

While Dr. Rush was concerned about excessive masturbation in the early nineteenth century, masturbation addiction as a disease or disorder didn't become a pop psychology phenomenon until the latter half of the twentieth century. The absence of almost two hundred years of medical opinion on masturbation addiction stemmed not only from the taboo against conducting research to better understand sexual behavior, but also from the unquestioned prevailing belief that masturbation in and of itself is a disease, regardless of whether a person was masturbating once a month or once an hour. But as masturbation became more normalized with the sexual revolution of the 1960s and '70s, a distinction started being made between healthy masturbation and addiction; a critical number of orgasms that indicates that you are compulsively engaging in self-abuse and giving into masturbatory

---

26. I spoke with mathematicians at my university and they assured me that this isn't true.

desires that will damage your health, end your relationships, and disappoint your pastor.

However, this distinction between healthy masturbation and masturbation addiction was often (and often still is) arbitrary. Its distinction is determined less by empirical evidence and more by ideological beliefs, reactionary politics, and fads within the mental health field. As was the case with the dawn of the Reagan-era and when Dr. Patrick Carnes popularized the term *sexual addiction* in his 1983 book, *Out of the Shadows* (originally and unimaginatively titled *The Sexual Addiction*). In his book, Dr. Carnes characterized high-frequency sexual desire and behaviors as an addiction, similar to addiction to substances like alcohol, cocaine, and heroin. Treatment, therefore, was modeled after drug rehabilitation clinics and popular 12-step programs like Alcoholics Anonymous. Just admit you touch yourself too much and turn your genitals over to a higher power.

Dr. Carnes has spent the last forty years hyper-focused on convincing the world that masturbation can be addicting. In a 2010 interview, he warned listeners about the apocalyptic dangers of masturbating to online pornography, saying, "We have a tsunami coming; a change in sexual behavior that's going to take us a hundred years to see what it does to the species." His life's work has spawned outpatient therapy practices, residential treatment facilities, addiction screening tests, self-help books, a professional organization for sex-addiction therapists, and a certification program for aspiring clinicians to specialize in sex addiction. It's almost as if he's addicted to promoting the concept of masturbation addiction.

Dr. Carnes, who earned his doctorate in counseling education from the University of Minnesota, believes masturbatory orgasm acts much like substance intoxication. Along with Dr. Drew, he is part of a cohort in the psychological and medical fields who are convinced that

Dr. Carnes's Assessment Tools

Dr. Carnes's assessment tools include the Sex Addiction Screening Test (SAST). It's freely and widely circulated online, primarily by anti-porn websites and addiction treatment centers. You can take the quiz yourself and realize just how much of a problem you have with touching yourself. Here are a few sample questions from the test for you to answer:

- Do you feel that your sexual behavior is not normal?
- Do you hide some of your sexual behaviors from others?
- Has sex (or romantic fantasies) been a way for you to escape your problems?
- Have you used the internet to make romantic or erotic connections with people online?
- Have you subscribed to sexually explicit materials?
- Have you spent considerable time surfing pornography online?

If you answered yes to all of these questions, according to the SAST, you may be a sex addict and should speak with a therapist. Other questions on this survey ask about BDSM, cruising and other public sex, having multiple partners, and engaging in sex work, all indicating that relationships and sexual behaviors that deviate from what is depicted on an episode of *Growing Pains* are signs of an addiction.

masturbation addiction is a real disease and are amply supplied with anecdotes about how masturbating too much is a destroyer of bodies, relationships, and souls. In unsolicited graphic detail, they will tell you how a patient's penis or clitoris doesn't work anymore because they spent too many hours masturbating with a Pringles can while watching pirate pegging porn.

On the other side of the debate are professionals like Dr. David Ley, a clinical psychologist and author of *The Myth of Sex Addiction*, who believe masturbation addiction is a made-up concept, typically used as an excuse for unethical (or even illegal) behavior and to over-pathologize normal sexual desires. From this perspective, those who get caught violating the boundaries of a relationship by masturbating to porn have to conveniently repent by admitting the "addiction," going to rehab as punishment to experience fifteen minutes of shame, and reemerging atoned of sexual sins and vowing never to transgress from their rigid, self-imposed sexual boundaries again.[27]

This position is argued largely because masturbation by itself and masturbation with porn do not act like addictive behaviors. Research does not support the contention that its mechanisms are similar to those of other addictive disorders, primarily due to a lack of tolerance and withdrawal symptoms. No masturbator, regardless of frequency, has to physically "detox" from their habit.

Critics of the concept that someone can become addicted to masturbation often point to the lack of any diagnosis listed in the *DSM* that would reflect or confirm this concept. Although there was a strong push to get Hypersexuality Disorder included in the *DSM-5* in 2013, which would have been an umbrella term that included excessive masturbation, the efforts ultimately failed due to a lack of empirical evidence

---

27. They'll transgress again.

supporting its inclusion as a mental disorder. Early drafts of the proposed criteria for Hypersexuality Disorder attempted to quantify the frequency of excessive orgasms by asserting that having an average of seven or more orgasms a week for at least six months would be hypersexual.

Seven a week.

This suggests that a daily masturbator would meet at least the frequency criterion of being a masturbation addict.

Dr. Martin Kafka, a clinical associate professor at Harvard Medical School and an advocate for the inclusion of Hypersexuality Disorder in the *DSM*, has argued that "by calling [high-frequency masturbation] an illness, you could be quite relieved that for something you have not really been able to control on your own, help is available." He adds that for someone who has been labeled a "scoundrel" by society, reframing the issue as a medical condition could help lead the individual to seek medical treatment.

Unsure if anyone has been called a "scoundrel" since the 1920s, Dr. Allen Frances, who is a professor emeritus of psychiatry at Duke University, believes Hypersexuality Disorder would be "wildly misapplied" and would over-pathologize normal sexual behaviors. When asked what he thought about the possibility of its inclusion in the *DSM*, Dr. Frances bluntly stated it would be "a really stupid idea."

The debate over whether masturbation addiction is real is not about whether someone can engage in masturbation unhealthily. No one argues that masturbation cannot lead someone to feel distress, shame, or out of control. The debate is more about what is causing unhealthy behavior, what to call it, and how to treat it.

Complicating matters is the fact that excessive masturbation can be a symptom of something else like a manic episode, stimulant intoxication, an anxiety or mood disorder, ADHD, or frontal lobe disinhibition caused by Alzheimer's disease. The problem with the masturbation addiction theory is that it assumes that high-frequency masturbation is the result of neurochemical addiction to orgasm, and therefore requires chemical dependency treatment. It's a one-size-fits-all solution to a complex phenomenon.

Despite the lack of solid evidence for the existence of masturbation addiction, this hasn't stopped the mental health field from capitalizing on fears and ignorance by launching a multimillion-dollar industry to rid you of masturbating more than a sex addiction therapist approves.

The High Cost of Masturbation Abstinence

A simple Google search for masturbation addiction yields thousands of blog posts and treatment programs aimed at curing a distressed person of their self-pleasure ailments. Dr. Carnes's residential treatment facility, Gentle Path at The Meadows, located on a thirty-five-acre compound fifty miles southwest of Phoenix, Arizona, is one such program that offers solitude away from solo sex. Residents of the facility are secluded for a whopping forty-five days without personal cell phones and computers, and engage in individual and group therapy with the aim of reducing masturbation frequency. So instead of masturbating for eight hours a day, you can go to therapy for eight hours a day.

Although personal electronic devices are banned from the facility (or at least confiscated upon admission) and no visitors are permitted for the entirety of the forty-five days, residents do have access to a landline telephone to occasionally speak with family members to update them on their treatment. When I spoke with a Gentle Path customer service representative about their phone policy, they could not confirm or deny a resident's ability to sneak a phone sex session in between therapy sessions.

Amenities at Gentle Path include facilities and activities that one would find at a nudist resort like a pool, sand volleyball, a putting green, and ping-pong tables. Mealtimes are prepared by their "Fuel Well" program to ensure healthy eating on your road to masturbation recovery. There are opportunities to partake in yoga and tai chi, take a stroll through the "serenity orchard," and stop in the "brain center."[28] There is also a labyrinth on the property grounds for masturbation addicts interested in re-creating the final scene in *The Shining*.

Since Gentle Path focuses on holistic healing, residents are able to express themselves artistically during art therapy sessions. Residents are offered an array of materials and mediums like paint and colored pencils to get creative in their treatment. It is unclear what the punishment would be for painting a nude Mona Lisa.

I'd imagine for most people, it would be difficult to afford the ability to put life on hold and step away from work and home responsibilities for forty-five days. However, some may argue that you can't put a price on recovery from masturbation addiction. For Gentle Path, that price is an all-inclusive $69,950. At almost seventy grand to alleviate masturbation distress, suddenly having a no-cost orgasm while looking at beautiful people on Instagram doesn't seem so distressing.

Even if someone could afford the time and money it takes to undergo intensive treatment to reduce masturbatory urges, is the treatment even effective? Dr. Joshua Grubbs, associate professor of psychology at the University of New Mexico, conducted a systematic review of twenty-five years of scientific literature on sex addiction, published between 1995 and 2020. The results of the review included 371 papers detailing 415 studies. Of these, only fifteen were focused on treatment, and of those, only three were randomized, controlled treatment studies,

---

28. Activities at the "brain center" were undisclosed on Gentle Path's website, so we are left to speculate whether they consist of Sudoku puzzles or lobotomies.

which is considered the gold standard in determining whether a particular treatment is effective.

Three studies.

In twenty-five years.

While these three studies show some promise utilizing either acceptance commitment therapy, cognitive behavioral therapy, or the antidepressant citalopram, three studies is far from conclusive in determining the best treatment approach for those believed to have an addiction to masturbation.

Of note, too, is the lack of research showing effectiveness in treating perceived excessive masturbation by having the patient attend 12-step groups or undergo long-term residential interventions as if they had an addictive disorder. In one study that surveyed former patients of a residential clinic in Canada, 71 percent of the respondents indicated some form of "relapse" of their sexual addiction after being discharged from a month-long inpatient treatment program. Whether it's twenty-one days at Dr. Drew's reality TV funhouse or forty-five days at Dr. Carnes's Wi-Fi-free desert oasis, there is simply no evidence to support that locking yourself away in a nunnery for a month will change how, when, or why you masturbate.

One of the problems with this body of literature on masturbation addiction is the inconsistent and imprecise measurement. Since there is no agreed-upon universal, operational definition of masturbation addiction, studies examining the topic have measured it in varied ways, making cross-study comparisons difficult and even impossible. Furthermore, masturbation addiction is most likely lumped under the general umbrella of sex addiction or porn addiction, and so it is unclear if the studies are actually measuring the effects of excessive masturbation or some other variable. Even after twenty-five years of research and 417 studies, what we know conclusively about masturbation addiction and its treatment can be summed up with a shrugging emoji.

I Think I Am Addicted, Therefore I Am

With ambiguity surrounding its diagnosis and a lack of evidence show-ing treatment effectiveness, how is it possible that so many people are convinced they are masturbation addicts? In a 2018 study in the United States, 10.3 percent of men and 7.0 percent of women reported at least occasionally feeling distressed over their sexual behavior, impulses, or desires. Studies from 2019 and 2020, also in the United States, found between 11 percent and 18.3 percent of men and between 3 percent and 4.7 percent of women who "somewhat agree" that they are addicted to pornography. In Poland in 2020, a study found similar findings, with 8.7 percent of men and 3 percent of women thinking they are at least somewhat addicted to porn. In Australia in 2017, the prevalence was slightly lower with 4.4 percent of men and 1.2 percent of women believ-ing they are porn addicts.

Priests, pastors, imams, and rabbis have spent centuries trying to convince us that touching our genitals disappoints God and goes against our "natural" purpose of genital function and use. It is no surprise, then, when a significant portion of the population internalizes these mes-sages and feels guilt and shame after masturbating. So much so that they vow never to touch themselves again, only to inevitably succumb to the temptations of the flesh and feel as if they have no control over their sexual desires.

Over the past decade, Dr. Grubbs and colleagues have repeatedly demonstrated that perceived problems related to one's sex life, espe-cially as it relates to masturbation and porn use, is predicted by a con-flict between one's sexual values and one's sexual behaviors. Termed *moral incongruence,* this theory posits that if a particular sexual behavior like masturbating or masturbating while watching porn goes against a person's moral or religious beliefs, but the person still engages in that behavior, they are likely to be distressed about the behavior. This distress cycle is interpreted as being out of control, and one is more likely to label themselves a sex addict as a result.

It is important to note that this phenomenon is not dependent on the frequency of masturbation. Even if someone's frequency is greater than average, that does not mean it is inherently excessive or a sign of a disorder. Someone could masturbate six times a day while thinking about Satanic sex orgies and be healthier than someone who masturbates just once a month while thinking about their wedding night.

Moral incongruence explains why. If someone has no qualms about masturbation—they believe it is perfectly normal and healthy to do it, regardless of the frequency—that person is unlikely to experience distress after masturbating. If they are in a relationship with a partner who feels similarly, then masturbation will unlikely cause relationship conflict. If they are efficient with masturbation, those six orgasms a day may only occupy less than an hour of the person's time and are unlikely to interfere with their other daily responsibilities.

But for the person who believes masturbation is unhealthy or a sin, vows never to masturbate, and/or is in a relationship in which their partner believes masturbating is equivalent to cheating, then even masturbating once a month is going to be a problem. The person will feel addicted because they swore they would abstain from the behavior but couldn't resist the urge. They will feel out of control because masturbating just once in a month is something they didn't want to do. They will feel guilty, anxious, or depressed afterward. If their partner finds out, a relational conflict ensues.

This demonstrates that problematic masturbation is not about masturbation per se or how often someone engages in it, but someone's values about masturbation and whether or not their masturbatory behavior aligns with those masturbatory values. They may be convinced that they have a sex problem because they've labeled themselves a masturbation addict. But if their religion prohibits them from masturbating, and they do it anyway and feel addicted as a result, that's not a sex problem; that's a religious problem.

Coming and Coping

In the rare case where someone's masturbation problems do not arise from moral incongruence, there is also concern over those who use masturbation as a way to regulate their mood, emotions, or stress.

Dr. Trish Leigh, a "certified brain health coach"[29] and staunch anti-porn advocate, believes that healthy masturbation is scheduled, not used for stress management or mood regulation, and must be void of sexual fantasies. So while you are staring at the wall during your scheduled 2 p.m. masturbation session, you must also make sure you are lacking any negative feelings that an orgasm would temporarily soothe.

Aside from the dubious credentials, Dr. Leigh's advice isn't fringe. It is a relatively common assertion that masturbation shouldn't be used for stress management or to regulate one's emotions. Doing so would be indicative of poor coping mechanisms and using an orgasm for "not the right reasons." Under this logic, relaxing with a novel in the tub is acceptable self-care for stress, but once you reach for the shower head to put the stream on your clitoris, somehow self-care turns into self-abuse.

---

29. It is not clear what this actually is, but I did discover that for $997, you can take an online course at Amen University to become a certified brain health coach.

A more nuanced assertion is to suggest that masturbation shouldn't be your *only* source of emotional regulation. This makes practical sense when you consider that we're likely to feel stressed in situations in which masturbation would not be an option to engage in to self-soothe. In order to avoid getting arrested for public indecency in a long line at the DMV, it is wise for us to have a variety of techniques to employ in times of stress that are situationally appropriate.

However, focusing solely on masturbation frequency or its use to regulate emotions as a sign of a problem in and of itself ignores the function of the behavior. For example, say someone is distressed that they are masturbating two hours a day to cope with anxiety and stress. They enter therapy with the goal of reducing that amount or eliminating it altogether. If they're just viewing masturbation as the problem, therapy will address how to replace masturbation with other coping strategies, like going for a walk, watching favorite shows on Netflix, or deep breathing. Treatment would be considered successful if the person is now masturbating for only fifteen minutes a day, and the remaining hour and forty-five minutes is spent on other self-care activities.

What's missing from this treatment is an acknowledgment of the need to have a coping mechanism, any coping mechanism, for two hours a day to deal with stress or anxiety. The root causes of the distress weren't addressed, but the coping mechanism was. This approach over-pathologizes masturbation, ignores its function, and attempts to modify a behavioral response to increase "acceptable" coping strategies.

All the yoga poses in the world won't alleviate the crushing stress people have from work, relationship conflicts, and family responsibilities. Does it matter what techniques you're using if they're effective at temporarily easing your anxiety? Is masturbation the problem or is the problem your stressful and unfulfilling job? Something to ponder and to discuss with your boss during your next quarterly review.

Do No Harm

The Dr. Drews and the Dr. Carnes of the world rarely focus on this nuanced approach to masturbatory health because it doesn't fit within their addiction model. When someone struggles with heroin use, most chemical dependency counselors don't strategize ways for the patient to use heroin healthily. So, when someone shows up to a sex addiction therapist's office with a self-diagnosis of masturbation addiction, treatment will logically focus on abstinence. At best, it would define "healthy masturbation" in some valued-laden way that would only have the person masturbating while listening to Enya and thinking about making love to their soulmate.

Even before "sex addiction" became a pop psychology phenomenon in the 1980s, the mental health field already demonstrated that it has a long history of over-pathologizing sexual behavior that deviates from what can be shown in a Hallmark Christmas movie. From queer sexualities to BDSM to sex work, therapists have been quick to assume, based on their own sexual ignorance and shame, that any sexual behavior that deviates from cisgender, heterosexual, penile-vaginal intercourse is inherently a cause or a consequence of a mental disorder. And although there has been a concerted effort over the past few decades to increase therapist competency surrounding diverse sexualities, therapist bias still exists.

Take, for example, Dr. Kafka's original frequency criterion of sex addiction that suggested one orgasm a day could be problematic. For the biased therapist, how would having sex with your spouse every day be viewed, compared to having sex with yourself every day? Daily sex with a spouse would be viewed as a very healthy and active sex life within a marriage. Masturbating every day brings up assumptions that the person is lonely, isolated, compulsive, unhealthily coping with stressors, and/or addicted.

It is also important for therapists to be critical of a patient's desire to modify a behavior without first examining the factors influencing that desire. In the case of perceived excessive masturbation and porn watching, even if the distress is solely caused by the person's religious beliefs that disapprove of the behavior, it would be easy for a patient to enter therapy with this complaint and for the therapist to go along with the patient's desire to decrease or eliminate masturbating to porn.

However, what if that same therapist had a patient who was a Southern Baptist who went out dancing with her secular friends? While the behavior is fun and relaxing, it also causes a lot of guilt, distress, and conflicts because dancing in clubs goes against her religious beliefs. If she came to therapy saying that she wants to dance less or stop dancing altogether, should the therapist automatically go along with that treatment goal? Or should they explore whether her religious values and prohibitions are undermining her authentic self?

I'd imagine in this thinly veiled *Footloose* example, it would be the latter. But why don't therapists approach a desire to stop masturbating because of religious prohibitions with the same skepticism? When religion and masturbation collide, why is masturbation, not religion, always viewed as the problem?

This debate over masturbation is muddied by the language war. Clearly, people's masturbation habits can be a problem in their life. But the public doesn't need to get involved in the clinical debate over whether those problems are reflective of an addiction, compulsion, impulsivity, or merely a symptom of something else. Instead, it is more valuable to expose the double standards surrounding the reasons that someone is concerned about their masturbation in the first place.

Going back to the previous Satanic sex orgy fantasy example, let's say someone was masturbating six times a day. Granted, six times per day is more than most people's masturbatory frequency, but so is running six miles a day, eating six servings of leafy vegetables, and teaching six senior citizens nude yoga. More doesn't always mean unhealthy.

If the duration is the concern, even if it took the person ten minutes to reach orgasm each time they masturbated, the six-times-a-day self-pleasurer would only be spending an hour with their hands on their genitals. Again, that is a longer duration than most people, but it's only an hour. There are twenty-three other hours in the day devoted to not masturbating. Ask yourself, How many hours a day do you spend watching shows on one of the dozen streaming services you subscribe to? How many hours do you spend just *scrolling* through the titles on those streaming services? Nobody is entering therapy or losing a relationship over a Disney+ addiction.

Aside from religious shame, much of the guilt surrounding the frequency of masturbation is the result of feeling as if you should have been doing something more constructive with your time. This is one of the central beliefs of masturbation abstainers. Known as "sexual sublimation," this approach among abstainers holds that the energy expended during masturbation could have been used for other pursuits. If only you didn't masturbate a few times a week while in college, you could have made the *Forbes'* 30 Under 30 list.

Masturbation is believed to be unhealthy because it is an opportunity cost. If you're masturbating, you're not doing other things. But everything is an opportunity cost. Spending time in the library studying for the LSAT is an opportunity cost to training for a marathon. Conversely, the time and energy it takes to train for a marathon could have been spent getting into law school. If you're so concerned that masturbating for a few minutes each week is somehow preventing you from becoming *Time* magazine's Person of the Year, there should be strong advocacy for not having children. What is a bigger time commitment and energy drainer than raising kids?

But therein lies the double standard and the subjectivity of what constitutes a noble use of your time and energy. If masturbation is devalued as juvenile, pathetic, or addictive, then you're going to feel guilty engaging in it and feel as though you should be spending your time doing something else. But if masturbation is valued as a brief sexual activity that is pleasurable and does no harm, then the few minutes a week touching yourself would be more respected and not scapegoated as the reason you're not raising capital and owning rockets.

Ironically, those who profess the benefits of sexual sublimation the loudest expend a lot of time and energy trying to convince others of the vital importance of conserving time and energy by not masturbating. It's almost as if their struggles to become a billionaire capitalist have nothing to do with how often they come.

But what about masturbating too much in a relationship? In my clinical experience, this was the most common scenario in which someone entered therapy over concerns about their masturbation. Typically, someone in a long-term, committed relationship got caught masturbating by their partner. They would often have ritualistic masturbation; not ritualistic like lighting black candles and ejaculating onto an altar, but ritualistic in the sense that they would wait for their family to go to bed, log onto the family computer, watch porn and masturbate, delete the browser history, and fall asleep.

Aside from guilt, this ritual was working for them in fulfilling sexual and emotional needs. That is until they got sloppy and fell asleep at the computer with bathhouseblowjobs.com on the screen only to be woken up by a very upset spouse the next morning.

Understandably, the discovering partner would have feelings of betrayal, confusion, anger, insecurity, and disgust. It tore the trusting foundation of the relationship. But instead of going into couples therapy to address the betrayal, along with the underlying reasons that fueled the secrecy, the nightly masturbator would self-diagnose as a masturbation/porn/sex addict and seek individual therapy to rid himself of the urge to ever touch his penis again.

All of this could have been prevented by having a conversation before the secrecy began about the role of masturbation in the relationship. There are those who disapprove of their partner masturbating, believing it is a form of cheating, and/or believing it is their responsibility to meet all of their partner's sexual needs. Although I could ideologically argue with the absurdity of that belief and assert that it is setting the relationship up for disaster, I don't dictate the sexual boundaries within others' relationships. If two people agree to this belief, have fun (or not).

But what shows up in therapy is when this belief is held only by one partner and reluctantly agreed to by the other. The person feels an "out-of-control" urge to masturbate despite it being prohibited in his relationship. For the therapist with anti-masturbation attitudes, the focus of treatment will be to strategize ways to manage this urge and to honor the relationship agreement.

To expose the double standard that exists with this abstinence approach, what if instead of a prohibition on masturbation and porn, there was a prohibition on golf? A person is not allowed to play golf or watch it on TV because their spouse forbids it. Would a therapist, or anyone for that matter, automatically believe that was a reasonable request and unquestionably support its enforcement?

But golf can be a source of distancing and conflict in a relationship. It takes a partner away from the house for hours at a time, often on weekends and holidays, when that time could be spent on joint activities with a partner. Golf also can cost a lot of money. Equipment and course fees or membership dues can be a financial burden for the couple, when that money could be spent on things or activities that benefit the relationship.

The difference is that we view golf as an acceptable hobby within a relationship and masturbating to porn as a dysfunctional activity within a relationship. It would be viewed as controlling to prohibit a partner from enjoying a round of golf on Saturdays, but an act of love for the relationship to prohibit them from masturbating.

I'm not denying that masturbation can't be a source of great pain in someone's life or relationship. I'm not dismissive of the stories people tell where they believe masturbation ruined their life in some capacity. What I am critical of, however, is how these issues are being talked about and how they are being treated, by both laypeople and mental health providers.

Because the reality is you're probably not masturbating too much. You're unlikely to have the neurological mechanisms of masturbation addiction. You're probably just fine.

So instead of pathologizing your masturbation frequency, what would happen if you simply accepted it? Without judgment. Accepted it and the elf porn that you're watching as a brief moment of pleasure and went on with your day. Because if there is one area of research that we can speak more definitively from, it's that if you think masturbation will be healthy for you, it likely will be.

CHAPTER 5

This Is Your Brain on Porn Illiteracy

Fight the New Drug, Porn Research, and Antisemitic Conspiracy Theories

The billboards erected across the San Francisco Bay Area in 2015 were hard to miss, even though they displayed a simple message: "Porn Kills Love." The tagline was part of a campaign orchestrated by the nonprofit Fight the New Drug, which was founded in 2009. Their mission is to communicate to the public the harmful effects of pornography using "science, facts, and personal stories" and to sell "Porn Kills Love" T-shirts so you can be the weirdo sporting prudish apparel at your company's annual potluck picnic.

Fight the New Drug is grounded in the belief that porn use is analogous to drug use, and that no amount or type of porn viewing can be healthy for a consumer. The group regularly gives lectures to schools and youth organizations that are probably as interesting and effective as DARE programming was during the height of the war on drugs.

Based out of Salt Lake City, Fight the New Drug claims to be a non-religious and non-legislative organization. And on the surface, that is true. The website is devoid of any overt proselytizing and religious messaging. There are no calls to action to ban porn in the name of Jesus or to embarrassingly picket outside of a Hustler Hollywood.

However, the organization's president and cofounder is Clay Olsen. Olsen is a former youth counselor for Especially for Youth, which is a summer camp to "strengthen youth in their commitment to live the gospel of Jesus Christ." He is also a current board member of the Utah Coalition Against Pornography, which cowrote a resolution for the Utah legislature declaring pornography a public health crisis—the first state to do so in the United States when it passed in 2016. Olsen spoke at the ceremonial signing of the resolution, calling the moment "historic" and a step in the right direction.

So even though Fight the New Drug is not overtly religious or legislative, it is situated within the context of Mormon theocracy. It is from within this context that Fight the New Drug creates a narrative that watching porn is inherently harmful to individuals, couples, and society. And they are certainly not alone in this fight against the alleged depravity of masturbating in front of a computer screen. They are joined by other religious moralists, self-identified male feminists, and white supremacists, all of whom are dedicated to eradicating the world of porn by making misleading claims over the effects of masturbating to such cinematic classics like *Anal Invaders 9: The Butt from Another Planet*.[30]

For Better, For Worse, For Richer, For Porno

When the "Porn Kills Love" campaign launched, I'm assuming Bay Area motorists were slightly confused by the ominous, yet cryptic billboards they passed on their commutes. "Porn kills love? How? Why? Does that include feet pics?"

Fight the New Drug asserts that humans are "hardwired" to need love and connection, and that masturbating while watching porn disrupts this need by making a sexual outlet free from effort and reciprocity.

---

30. *Anal Invaders 9: The Butt from Another Planet* (also known as *They Came from Planet Butt*) was nominated for two Adult Video News awards in 1996, winning Best Anal–Themed Feature. This trivia makes for excellent small talk at wedding receptions.

They describe it as "counterfeit intimacy" that will destroy relationships and will have you quickly hiring a divorce attorney to argue over custody of the family guinea pig.

To Fight the New Drug's credit, there is a considerable amount of research that has demonstrated a consistent association between men's self-reported porn use and being dissatisfied in their romantic and sexual relationships. Further, in a large sample of heterosexual women, the more they believed their husbands watched porn, the lower the quality they reported in their relationship.

At face value, this might suggest that porn does, indeed, kill love. A husband's browser history of "big-tittied goth girlfriends" could warrant a session with a marriage therapist. However, the association between porn and relational satisfaction exists bi-directionally, meaning that as men become increasingly dissatisfied in their relationships, they tend to watch porn. In turn, the more they watch porn, the more dissatisfied they become in their relationships. Longitudinal studies testing the origin of this association fail to show the chicken (porn use) coming before the egg (dissatisfaction).

Interestingly, too, this relationship does not exist for women, and some studies even show that the more porn women watch, the more satisfied they are in their relationships. And while a few studies have shown associations between a partner's porn use and relationship satisfaction, an equal number of studies have found no correlation, suggesting that the amount of porn a partner uses in a relationship doesn't always predict the relationship quality for the other partner.

Complicating matters more is the role of other variables that may better explain the observed relationships (when they exist) between porn use and relationship satisfaction. Sociologists Dr. Samuel Perry and Dr. Andrew Whitehead found a negative relationship between porn viewing and sexual satisfaction for men (but not women), but when they factored in religiosity (as measured by church attendance and opinion about the Bible) the association only remained for the believers. This supports the moral incongruence theory, holding that those who believe porn is unhealthy and try to abstain from it are more likely to experience negative effects when watching it than those who have more positive attitudes toward porn.

More so, in a separate study by Dr. Perry, he found that the relationship between porn use and poor relationship quality disappeared when accounting for masturbation, suggesting that solo sex should be examined as the active ingredient in influencing relationship quality and not porn use in and of itself.

While there is some consistency in the research finding an association between men's self-reported porn use and poor relationship satisfaction, this relationship is challenged by the presence of moral incongruence and the directionality of the relationship. And although there is probably an anecdote out there about how a marriage was ended by someone finding their spouse's stash of Viking porn,[31] the claim that porn kills love is unsupported.

Armchair Neuroscientists

One of the top assertions Fight the New Drug makes is that masturbating to porn affects the viewer like a drug by literally changing the structure and the function of the brain. Fight the New Drug is savvy in that they have put together a website that, on the surface, seems to make a compelling argument that masturbating to porn is inherently harmful. They cite dozens of scientific sources to back up their claims and

---

31. Being a resident of Minnesota, I am required by state law to make a reference to Vikings, lakes, Prince, or the phrase "you betcha!" at least once in every publication.

provide countless links to learn more about various topics relating to porn science and the harms of masturbating to porn.

However, a closer look at their claims will reveal a smoke-and-mirrors show that lacks any real substance. For example, in their article on how porn changes the brain, they review several studies about neural pathways of addiction, neuroplasticity, and neurological imaging showing brain structure differences. A total of thirty-six references are cited throughout the article, making the case that porn use changes our brains, chemically, neurologically, and structurally.

But within the list of thirty-six references, it is easy to note that many are duplicates. There are only thirteen distinctive articles that are referenced. Of those, only six are about sex, and of those, only four are specifically about porn and the brain. None of the four studies were methodologically designed to test whether porn *causes* any brain changes. At best, two of the studies used an MRI to examine brain structural and functional differences in the participants, and correlated the differences with the participants' self-reported pornography use. This suggests an association between porn use and the measured neurological differences, not a causal relationship.[32]

One of the most frequently cited research articles that claims to have identified an association between porn consumption and brain damage is a 2014 article published in *JAMA Psychiatry*. The study included sixty-four German men whose brains were scanned using an MRI. The results showed that as self-reported pornography use increased, the volume of the participants' gray matter in the right caudate nucleus of the brain decreased. This part of the brain is responsible for a number of important functions, including learning, planning, and memory. The

---

32. If you remember anything from a research methods or statistics class in college, it is hopefully that correlation does not equal causation.

results from the study are certainly interesting, and they might suggest that porn use does in fact change the gray matter in the brain. However, it could also mean that lower volume of gray matter makes porn more enjoyable or rewarding to watch. Or it could mean that there is some other unidentified variable that is having an impact on both porn use and gray matter. This study does not allow us to state any of those possibilities with certainty.

While the direction of this relationship is uncertain, the more important limitation is that all the men in the study, regardless of the amount of porn consumed and brain differences observed by the MRI, were healthy and without functioning impairments. In the real world, people don't get MRIs without symptoms,[33] making any neuroimaging findings practically useless on their own.

And even if the study utilized random assignment and exposed half of the participants to porn and the other half to non-sexual media and then subsequently measured their gray matter volume, one study involving sixty-four men would not allow us to make the definitive statement that porn use changes the brain. Like all science, the study would need to be replicated with larger and more diverse samples to better understand the active ingredients that are contributing to the observed differences. A single study will never give us definitive answers. It is just one piece of a sexually explicit puzzle.

Other studies on the relationship between porn viewing and brain functioning are equally complex and misunderstood. In 2017, researchers examined brain differences between compulsive porn users and healthy controls and found no differences when shown erotic images, but significant differences when cued for erotic images, suggesting that

---

33. And without prior authorization from an American health insurance company that may also require a blood sacrifice.

compulsive porn users are more activated at the *prospect* of seeing porn. This might be a conditioning effect, meaning that compulsive porn users become more activated when around objects that remind them of watching porn, like computers and boxes of Kleenex.

While there is some support for compulsive porn use being associated with different neurological functioning, compared to those who are not compulsive, few conclusions can be drawn about the effects of porn use on the brain.

Hypothetically, let's say Fight the New Drug was correct in their assertion that watching porn unequivocally changes the brain. What anti-porn advocates fail to report is that many behaviors that are pleasurable and done repeatedly can cause changes in the brain. This would include watching porn, riding bikes, playing the piano, having kids, and praying the rosary. But, unsurprisingly, Fight the New Drug does not express concern over the neurological changes from taking your kids to church.

I Am a Male Feminist, Hear Me Roar

Covert Mormon organizations are not the only anti-porn groups trying to regulate and police what you watch while you masturbate. Feminists and feminist organizations have a long history of debating whether pornography is healthy for women, culminating in the "pornography wars" of the 1970s and '80s. Some feminists like Betty Dodson and Annie Sprinkle believe pornography is a form of sexual freedom of expression and represents bodily autonomy, for both the porn performer and the viewer. Other feminists like Andrea Dworkin and Dr. Gail Dines argue that pornography is filmed violence against women that perpetuates rape culture and the objectification of women by men.

Unsurprisingly, male academics have inserted themselves (and often centered themselves) in this feminist ideological debate like self-identified radical feminist Dr. Robert Jensen. Aside from arguing about why trans women should not be allowed in women's restrooms and why drag shows are misogynistic, Dr. Jensen has spent much of his career arguing on behalf of women about what is best for them as it relates to porn.

As a professor emeritus in the School of Journalism and Media at the University of Texas at Austin, Dr. Jensen has written extensively on why pornography promotes violence against women. He has argued that men who enjoy watching double penetration porn videos, for example, are sadistically aroused by the image of a woman being penetrated by two men because they know no woman could ever enjoy that behavior. He bases this argument on the fact that he has never personally met a woman who expressed interest in double penetration. This is not only an example of Dr. Jensen being creepy for asking his female friends if they fantasize about double penetration, but it's also an example of a logical fallacy and the need for Dr. Jensen to get a more sexually adventurous social network.

Although a staunch anti-porn advocate, noticeably absent from Dr. Jensen's writings is any mention of whether masturbation is healthy. And as neuroscientist Dr. Nicole Prause has argued in a published paper in *Archives of Sexual Behavior*, porn is for masturbation. From this argument, any discussion about the effects of porn cannot be teased apart from the effects of masturbation. To condemn porn, without specifying how masturbation in and of itself can be healthy, is to also condemn masturbation.

The feminist ideological debate about the effects of pornography on women is just that—ideological. It's often grounded in the belief that porn is harmful and then relies on mental masturbation to philosophically support the belief that watching porn is akin to abusing women.

The science, however, paints a different story.

A meta-analysis published in 2021 analyzed the findings from fifty-nine studies that examined the link between sexual aggression against women and pornography consumption among the general population. Results indicated no relationship between nonviolent porn use and sexual violence, especially long-term effects. And although watching violent porn was slightly predictive of sexual violence, the correlation disappeared when the analyses controlled for citation bias.[34] What porn use did predict was an increased risk of sexual violence recidivism for high-risk offenders. Unless you are already prohibited from living a thousand feet from a Chuck E. Cheese, watching porn will not make you a danger to your community.

The data on porn and sexual violence are complex and often show contradictory findings. Although there is some support for the assertion that watching violent porn is associated with an increased risk of violence (especially for those who have already committed sex offenses and are considered at high risk of recidivism), better predictors of violence against women include personality characteristics and traits such as callousness and hypermasculinity, as well as engagement in non-sexual deviant behavior. To say that masturbating while watching porn will lead someone to commit acts of sexual violence against women is an overgeneralization and a misrepresentation of the research.

Porn Power, Not White Power

Although ideologically opposed in most areas, conservative Mormons and anti-porn feminists are joined in their crusade against smut by a seemingly unlikely ally: white supremacists. In a 2018 blog post, David

---

34. *Citation bias* occurs when you heavily cite sources that support your hypotheses and results, while omitting sources that have found alternative results. For example, if your anti-vax uncle is trying to convince you that vaccines cause AIDS by only citing sources he's seen on the Facebook group MAGA FREEDOM MEN, he likely has a citation bias.

Duke, former Republican representative in the Louisiana state legislature and founder of the Knights of the Ku Klux Klan, stated, "When sick Jewish pornographers are part of the brutality of Jewish organized crime, the results can obviously be horrifically tragic for our people." Earlier in 2006, before Twitter permanently suspended his account for hate speech, Duke tweeted at porn star legend Jenna Jameson that "Jews dominate porn—why are 'Christians' ok with that?"

For Duke, and other white supremacists who think of themselves as exemplars of a "superior race," pornography isn't just immoral for violating sexual social norms. To them, porn is a Jewish conspiracy to degrade and weaken white men.

Dr. Kristoff Kerl, a postdoctoral fellow at the University of Copenhagen, reviewed this conspiracy theory in his article "Oppression by Orgasm: Pornography and Antisemitism in Far-Right Discourses in the United States Since the 1970s." According to the antisemitic conspiracy theories of white nationalists and supremacists, Jews create and distribute pornography to threaten the patriarchal sexual order of Western, white men. The order is threatened by destroying the sexual purity of white women and emasculating white men, which ultimately leads to the broader conspiracy theory of white genocide.

When porn depicts non-white men, especially in the form of interracial sex scenes, antisemites believe it increases white women's sexual desire for men of color and Jewish men. Antisemites fear this will result in white women procreating with other races and ultimately exterminating the future Aryan race.

Also, according to this illogical, racist theory, when white men watch porn, it makes them weak and docile. By turning men into "betas," porn prevents men from fighting for a white ethno state and will also make them less attractive to white women who value strong men with whom they can procreate and make racist babies.

In an unsurprising adjunct to this conspiracy, antisemites believe that watching porn can cause straight men to become gay. The theory posits that white men will get bored with watching the "sexual purity" of penile-vaginal intercourse and will have to seek out novel sexual depictions, like anal sex with men and sex with transgender women. And, again, the concern here is if all the white men turn gay, there will be fewer white offspring in the next generation to be paranoid about porn turning racists gay.

This is a common belief among non-racists, too, but there is no solid empirical evidence to support the assertion that viewing pornography acts like chemical dependency and creates physical tolerance, where the viewer will require "harder-core" images and videos in order to experience sexual arousal. Masturbating to a *Playboy* in your teens does not mean you're eventually going to need pornography depicting a man being flogged with an iguana in order to get off in adulthood.

Anti-porn and anti-masturbation attitudes are not new among the far right, with leaders of Hitler Youth warning young Germans about the dangers of non-procreative sexual behavior, including masturbation, in the 1930s. Today, the polo-clad and unintentionally homoerotically named Proud Boys, who believe that "West is best," encourage their members to abstain from porn and limit masturbation to once per month. Leaders of the small, pan-European identity fascist group in the United States, Patriot Front monitors and shames its members about their porn use. Nick Fuentes, a Gen-Z neo-Nazi and leader of the shitposting "Groyper Army," believes that "masturbation is gay." Far-right conspiracy theorist Paul Joseph Watson, when not ranting about chemtrails, tweeted in 2019, "Porn is evil. It literally re-wires your brain and causes erectile dysfunction. Take the pledge. Don't be a Coomer."[35]

---

35. A Coomer is internet slang for someone who excessively masturbates, especially to porn. The term is often accompanied by a "Wojak" meme of a balding, bearded man that, unfortunately but coincidentally, looks a lot like me.

The link between porn viewing and sexual dysfunction, especially erectile difficulties, is widely touted by religious moralists, anti-porn feminists, and white supremacists alike. But despite the few case reports of men blaming their erectile dysfunction on pornography (with the belief that they have become desensitized to porn images, and in-person sex can no longer compete), the available empirical evidence does not support this assertion. In a 2011 study published in 2015 involving thousands of European men, data were analyzed from two separate measures of erectile functioning and self-reported pornography use. In the first analysis, only Croatian men (not Norwegian or Portuguese) showed a small relationship between porn use and erectile ability. For these men, moderate porn use mildly predicted erectile problems. But interestingly, *heavy* porn use did *not* predict erectile dysfunction. In the second analysis, no relationship was found between any amount of porn use and erectile difficulties for any of the three nationalities.

In 2019, Dr. Grubbs and colleagues found no relationship between erectile difficulties and porn use among a US sample, but there was a relationship between sexual dysfunction and those who self-reported problematic porn use. However, there was no clear association from longitudinal analyses, which does not provide evidence to support the contention that porn use *caused* erectile problems over time, especially in men without self-reported porn problems.

A 2022 study in Austria found no relationship between porn use and sexual functioning problems for men (regardless of how realistic they thought porn was), but researchers found a positive relationship for women's porn use and sexual functioning via increased sexual flexibility. This suggests that porn use for women is associated with increased engagement in a variety of sexual behaviors, which, in turn, is associated with better sexual functioning.

"But this happened to me!" laments a reader of the Daily Stormer, who believes a daily dose of anime breasts was the reason he couldn't get it up and why his girlfriend cheated on him. The reality is the men who report this connection are likely overlooking other causal factors contributing to erectile dysfunction, such as anxiety, alcohol use, or trying to get aroused while in the refractory period after an orgasm.

Much like the insecure masculinity that drives semen retention, white supremacists scapegoat masturbating to porn to account for their own shortcomings. Since they feel as if they have so little control over why their life is miserable, they try to regulate and control their own bodies and the bodies of others. It is what cultural studies scholar Simon Strick refers to as the alt-right politics of self-help and self-improvement. You may not have a decent job, a girlfriend, or an ideal masculine physique, but at least you can pull yourself up by your Gestapo bootstraps and resist the urge to masturbate to porn.

What is fascinating about this porn paranoia by white supremacists is that they claim to be the "superior race." A race that is superior in terms of intellect and behavior. But, somehow this superiority can be overpowered by looking at pixelated nipples.

While it is easy to poke fun at tinfoil hat–wearing bigots who think they're winning a race war by not touching their own genitals, this hatred and conspiratorial thinking about Jews weaponizing porn to maim white men can have deadly outcomes. White supremacists have routinely harassed, doxed, and threatened employees and executives of the pornography tube site PornHub. Robert Bowers, who killed eleven Jews at a synagogue in Pittsburgh in 2018, was concerned about "Jewish porn bots" on social media before the slaughter. And white nationalist Anders Behring Breivik ranted about the moral decay caused by Judaism and porn before killing seventy-seven people in Norway in 2011.

So if you're a white person preoccupied with racist conspiracy theories about Jews trying to replace your race through porn, I want you to take a deep breath, go to therapy, and go fuck yourself.

A Research Dumpster Fire

Like clockwork, if I mention pornography on my social media accounts and do not fully condemn its existence and the harm it causes, an upset stranger will tell me to "do my research" and will provide a link to a study that doesn't make the argument they think it is making. I have been doing research on this topic for almost twenty years. But "doing research" also means having the scientific literacy to understand the research studies you're reading.

Unlike the false belief that vaccines cause autism, which was spawned by only two poorly designed studies and fueled misinformation for decades, there is not a small number of pseudoscientific studies on the negative effects of masturbating to porn that has generated years of fearmongering. Instead, it's almost *all* the research on porn since the 1970s that has either been poorly designed or misinterpreted and overgeneralized. Which is why Dr. Taylor Kohut, a research associate at Western University in Ontario, Canada, who has studied pornography for more than a decade, refers to the body of scientific literature on porn as "basically a dumpster fire."

One of the most significant problems regarding porn research is a lack of a universally accepted definition of what porn even is, as well as a lack of consistent ways to measure its use. Of all the studies on pornography published between 1999 and 2009, 95 percent used a unique, researcher-created definition of pornography. Further, 59 percent of the studies lacked clear reporting of how porn use was measured, and 10 percent provided no information at all.

THIS IS YOUR BRAIN ON PORN ILLITERACY

This lack of consistent measurement and use of a single definition of pornography makes cross-study comparisons difficult (if not impossible), and gives rise to questions about whether porn use is even being measured at all. For example, in a 2011 study on frat boys' use of porn and associated misogynistic attitudes, researchers asked college students whether they have recently seen "media consisting of sadomasochistic portrayals of bondage, whipping and spanking but without an explicit lack of consent in video, movies, magazines, books or online." Answering *yes* to this question could mean that the guy is watching fetish porn every day that depicts the use of anal hooks, cattle prods, and blood play. Or it could mean that he simply read a review of *50 Shades of Grey* in *Entertainment Weekly*.

Another methodological problem with porn research is the underlying assumption that porn is harmful in some way. Studies then are designed to test research hypotheses that predict negative effects or associations. This skews the published data on the topic to favor studies that have demonstrated such negative effects or associations, at the expense of ignoring neutral or positive outcomes from watching porn.

But one of the most concerning methodological flaws in pornography research is the fact that very few studies ask specific questions about the content of porn or report the content of the porn used in the experiment. Historically, porn is treated as a monolith within the social sciences, without any meaningful attempts to differentiate between behaviors depicted on camera. If we are concerned about porn effects, what are the effects from?

Porn is not much different from other media that is consumed regularly. Are we concerned about the gender role stereotypes and narrow standards of beauty in porn? How are those themes any different than what is depicted in Disney movies? If it's violence, aggression, and dominance that are concerning, the effects of horror movies should have been the focus of scientific examination over the past fifty years. If it's the nudity and sex that would lead to negative outcomes, wouldn't watching porn be no different than watching episodes of *Euphoria* or *Game of Thrones*?

The only significant pictorial or thematic difference between porn and other media is the explicitness of the sex. But that begs the question: Is seeing an erect penis go into a vagina such a powerful image that we would expect viewers to be forever altered in their relationships, behavior, and neurology? While some sexual narcissists may think the world revolves around their erection, a few inches of flesh is not that powerful.

The bigger difference is not about the content of porn but the motivation behind why we watch it. The primary motivation to watch porn is to aid in masturbation. Aside from a few fetishists, masturbation is not the main motivator for people to watch *Halloween* or *Finding Nemo*. Similar to the findings of Dr. Perry's research, "porn effects" may not be about porn at all, but about the role of masturbation in one's life.

This aligns with my former clinical work, where objections to porn use within relationships were actually about objections to masturbation. Whether there were beliefs that masturbation was cheating or insecurity about sexual needs getting met without a partner, secret masturbation was the actual cause of the distress, betrayal, and subsequent conflict. But it is a lot easier for couples to argue about porn use than to have a vulnerable conversation about privacy, boundaries, the role of masturbation in the relationship, desire discrepancies, and why one partner is aroused by clown feet.

After fifty years of porn research, few things can be said unequivocally about the impact of watching people have sex on film. Some evidence lends support to the contention that porn may not be the healthiest option for religious people who morally object to porn, partners who disapprove of their significant other watching porn, and high-risk sex offenders. But for the rest of us, as a whole, porn watching is likely to be inconsequential. It is simply a momentary experience to aid in self-inducing an orgasm.

The widespread concern about the effects of pornography is a moral panic rooted in conspiratorial thinking and scientific illiteracy. It is no different today than it was in the nineteenth century when Dr. Kellogg was gravely concerned about effects of "lewd stories."

Watching porn will not lead to the annihilation of a race. It will not make you dependent on Viagra. It will not damage your brain to the point of dysfunction. It can, however, be a medium to explore your sexuality more in depth to better know yourself. It can help facilitate the pleasure of masturbation and the goal of orgasm. And it is one of the few mediums where you can satisfy your fantasy of watching two nuns kissing.

CHAPTER 6

Know Thyself

Sex Therapy, Learning to Come, and Masturbation Explorers

Sexual revolutionary Betty Dodson had grown tired of the consciousness-raising groups that were popular during the women's rights movement in the 1970s. No longer desiring to sit in circles describing the horrors of misogyny, Dodson wanted to fight the patriarchy by creating a space where women could explore and celebrate solo sexuality. For Dodson, to liberate masturbation was to liberate women.

Working out of her own apartment in New York, she transformed her living room into a masturbatorium called the "Temple of Pleasure," complete with erotic art and mirrors lining the walls and plush carpet lining the floor. Atop the fireplace mantel hung a large photo of a completely nude Dodson striking a yoga pose.

Meeting weekly for a month, the newly formed "BodySex Workshops" started off with a small group of nude women discussing their bodies and learning about the mechanics and diversity of masturbation and orgasm from Dodson. The groups were open to all women, regardless of sexual orientation, relationship status, and age. To Dodson, these labels were of little importance to the liberation of masturbation. What was important was recognizing the group's shared identity of being sexual women.

Early on, the group was only led didactically with Dodson serving as the teacher and informing the attendees about masturbation and orgasm. She would assign masturbation as homework and had a box full of vibrators for attendees to borrow for their assignments. However, it wasn't long before the class moved from didactic to experiential, with women in attendance, particularly those who were unsure if they had ever experienced an orgasm, requesting that Dodson actually masturbate in class.

Dodson, not one to shy away from artistic expression, turned her instructive orgasms into a performance. She would first walk around the room mimicking women's expected timidity and passivity with sex, pretending to bashfully walk in high heels. Then she would flip the gender script and demonstrate how women could own and expand their space. She would encourage others to join in by "walking tall with our heads up, tits out, buttocks tucked under, and clits forward." Afterwards, Dodson would grab her vibrator and demonstrate what masturbation and orgasm could look like. Sometimes they were big orgasms with plenty of body spasms and vocalizations, whereas other times they were small and quiet. Dodson's modeling showed the women in attendance there's no right or wrong way to climax.

Dodson acknowledged that there wasn't really a women's equivalent to a men's "circle jerk," so when several attendees suggested they wanted to join in on the masturbation demonstrations, Dodson leapt at the opportunity. She lit a candle in the center of a circle of fifteen women to create a ritual space, and then all attendees pleasured themselves with fingers or vibrators to orgasm. Reflecting back on this experience in her book, *Sex for One*, Dodson recalled, "The combination of playing teacher, being a voyeur of the erotic sights, exhibiting my sexuality, and getting paid to masturbate to orgasm with all these wonderful women was hedonistic heaven beyond my wildest dreams."

Dodson wasn't alone in her mission to liberate masturbation. For decades, but especially during the sexual revolution of the 1960s and '70s, masturbation pioneers focused their energies on developing new therapies and techniques to aid those on a quest of a solo orgasm.

Learning to Come

Three years before Dodson was having masturbatory show-and-tell in her Temple of Pleasure, Dr. William Masters and Virginia Johnson, researchers at Washington University in St. Louis, published *Human Sexual Inadequacy*. The groundbreaking book included details about their studies on teaching women how to masturbate to overcome an inability to orgasm; a clinical intervention known, unpoetically, as *directed masturbation*.

Following Masters and Johnson's lead, psychology professor Dr. Joseph LoPiccolo and his graduate student at the time Charles Lobitz published a nine-step directed masturbation program in 1972 in the academic journal *Archives of Sexual Behavior*. Dr. Lonnie Barbach modified this program in 1974 to include a group treatment component referred to, un-euphemistically, as the "Preorgasmic Women's Group."[36]

By the end of these directed masturbation programs, there is a high likelihood that the formerly preorgasmic woman is now orgasmic. Since its inception in the 1970s, directed masturbation has been studied for its effectiveness, with 60 to 90 percent of women becoming orgasmic with masturbation and 33 to 85 percent becoming orgasmic with a partner.

When directed masturbation is used in a treatment program by a sex therapist, it is important to mention that the therapist is not showing

---

36. Preorgasmic doesn't mean the person is on the verge of having an orgasm. It's synonymous with anorgasmic, which means the person has never experienced an orgasm. Preorgasmic is intentional framing suggesting that the person is capable of climaxing, but is in the "before times."

the patient how to masturbate, and the patient is not masturbating in front of the therapist during the session. While that may have been the radical and effective approach utilized by Dodson, mental health licensing boards generally frown upon nudity in therapy.

The role of the therapist at the onset of a directed masturbation intervention is to simply describe the process, and for the patient to complete the exercises in the privacy of their own home. There are multiple steps completed over the course of as many weeks. In between these steps, the patient is meeting with the therapist to discuss what was effective and where they struggled. The therapy sessions are also an opportunity to focus treatment on other problems that may interfere with orgasm and pleasure like distracting thoughts, negative self-talk, poor body image, and sexual trauma.

There are several steps involved in directed masturbation, which focuses on increasing mindfulness of bodily sensations, including both non-sexual and sexual touch. Other steps deal with increasing knowledge about vulvar anatomy using a handheld mirror. Prior to the self-exploration at home, some therapists use session time discussing the differences between the labia minora and majora, the vestibule, the urethral and vaginal openings, the perineum, the mons pubis, and the clitoral hood and glans using diagrams or 3D models.[37] An added bonus of this step is gaining the ability to impress your friends by using the adjective *vulvar* in casual conversation.

Lastly, other steps of directed masturbation focus on the use of pornography, vibrators, and fantasy. A homework assignment may include writing a sex scene in a journal that has all the elements that you find

---

37. Some therapists use a plush vulva hand puppet when discussing sexual anatomy with their patients. I personally find using the puppets to be infantilizing because they look like a detached vulva from Snuffleupagus.

arousing: type of partner, behaviors to engage in, the ideal location and setting, and whether fantasy partners have their socks on or off.

Learning Not to Come

Given our culture's sexist expectations of female passivity, refusal to acknowledge female sexual desire, and reluctance to teach about the anatomy and function of clitorises, many women may struggle becoming orgasmic. Not seeking out self-help or clinical interventions like directed masturbation will often leave women reluctantly accepting not being able to orgasm.

For many men, though, they may have the opposite experience as preorgasmic women and are very skilled at reaching orgasm. So skilled, in fact, that they are able to climax in a matter of seconds compared to the more typical two to seven minutes. These efficient masturbators have learned exactly what type of stimulation their body craves and are able to become aroused and orgasm faster than it takes most people to toast an Eggo.

Within the masturbation realm, this isn't a problem. Throughout childhood and adolescence, many boys learn how to quickly (and silently) masturbate to orgasm to avoid detection from an intrusive parent or a nosy sibling. By the time they graduate from high school, these stealthy masturbators know their body so well they will be able to have an orgasm in under a minute in the college dorms without their pre-med roommate ever looking up from their biochem textbook.

This quickness is viewed as an asset. But this asset turns into a liability during their first college hookup when they repeat this rapid ejaculation during anal or vaginal intercourse with a new partner. Typically, the partner is desiring stimulation lasting longer than a few thrusts, so now the efficient masturbator is gaining the reputation on campus as being a "two-pump chump."

Clinically referred to as "premature ejaculation," the *DSM* defines this disorder as experiencing orgasm within sixty seconds of intercourse and before the person desires it. Everyone will likely experience rapid ejaculation at some point during their sexual history. If you haven't had sex in a while, and you are with a new partner, it is not surprising that sometimes in these scenarios your body quickly goes "Oh boy!" and you're left apologizing and lying to your partner that "this never happens."

Since numerous situations could make ejaculation "premature," the *DSM* requires the problem to occur during 75 to 100 percent of sexual encounters over the course of at least six months. Beyond the persistency and consistency of premature ejaculation, the most important criterion is that orgasm is happening before the person wants to. If someone ejaculates within fifteen seconds, and both partners are like "That's awesome; well done," then there is no distress. No distress means there's no premature ejaculation disorder, regardless of how fast the person comes.

Conversely, many patients enter therapy concerned about the timing of their orgasms, believing they are ejaculating too soon and certainly before they want to. Further assessment reveals that they are actually able to have intercourse for fifteen to twenty minutes before having an orgasm, but they desire to last more than an hour. In these scenarios, the focus of therapy is primarily educational, where the patient is informed about typical sexual responses and how the "going all night" myth violates the laws of friction.

But for those who are experiencing rapid ejaculation consistently with a partner and it is leading to sexual dissatisfaction, therapy focuses on another masturbation exercise developed by Masters and Johnson: the stop-start technique.

It is a misunderstanding about the physiology of orgasm to believe the best strategy to gain ejaculatory control is to distract yourself during sex by thinking about something dull like your grandpa's coin collection. Regardless of genitalia, orgasm is a spinal cord reflex. And while thoughts can help or hinder the sexual response, ultimately your body is perfectly capable of ejaculating while you're thinking about a 1936 buffalo nickel.

The key to gaining better ejaculatory control is to tune in to your bodily sensations, not to distract yourself from them. At its core, the stop-start technique is a series of steps designed to increase awareness of how your body is responding to sexual stimulation. By increasing awareness, you are able to make subtle adjustments to the stimulation to delay orgasm.

Like directed masturbation exercises, the stop-start technique is practiced by the patient alone and at home. In-session time is spent exploring what worked and what didn't, as well as addressing co-morbidities like anxiety and body image disturbances that may also be contributing to ejaculating prematurely.

Initial steps involve the patient masturbating without lubricant and without online pornography. A type of analog masturbation like you're a twelfth-century blacksmith. Once arousal increases moderately, whether that is in one second or one minute, masturbation stops. Hands off the penis completely like you're playing an obscene game of hot potato. Masturbation can resume once arousal decreases some, but some level of erection is maintained. This stopping and starting continues for at least fifteen minutes before allowing the ejaculation to occur and the celebrating to commence.

Later steps involve incorporating the use of lubricants, pornography, and sex toys like a masturbation sleeve (or for those with larger discretionary spending budgets, a RealDoll). This increases the sensation and makes it more challenging to control the timing of orgasm. Ultimately, the stopping and starting is replaced by slowing down, lightening the grip, or changing positions in order to slow the arousal.

This waxing and waning better mirrors what stimulation would be like during intercourse with a partner. It is more desirable to make small adjustments during intercourse like slowing down and changing positions, instead of just outright stopping, leaving your partner saying, "Again?"

Unfortunately, despite the stop-start technique being used as a gold standard sex therapy intervention for premature ejaculation, little evidence exists that it actually works by itself. Only two studies have shown that the stop-start method delayed ejaculation by 1.6 minutes (using a vibrating sex toy) and 7 minutes (without any sex toys). In three studies comparing the stop-start method to SSRI antidepressants,[38] SSRIs showed superiority to the masturbation treatment by delaying ejaculation by 1.22 to 3.55 minutes. In three other studies examining the stop-start method plus medication versus medication alone, all three studies favored the combination treatment with improvements in delaying orgasm from 30 to 60 seconds.

These treatment studies reflect a limitation in the diagnosis of premature ejaculation itself. Increasing time to reach orgasm doesn't necessarily mean decreasing distress about the timing of ejaculation. Other variables like pleasure and satisfaction are absent in these studies, as the focus is solely on the effects of treatment in increasing time until

---

38. SSRIs are notorious for causing sexual side effects, like delayed orgasm. For most people, this side effect is distressing and a common cause to discontinue the medication, even if it is helpful for anxiety or depression. However, for those with premature ejaculation, this side effect is welcomed with open arms.

ejaculation. While statistically significant, ninety seconds of additional thrusting isn't necessarily adding any pleasure or satisfaction.

Learning about the stop-start exercises, you may be thinking, *Isn't this just edging?*

Yes, yes it is.

Edging is the practice of masturbating close to the point of orgasm and then either stopping or slowing down in order to prolong the pleasure. Although edging is demonstrating ejaculatory control that may generalize to having sex with a partner, the goal of edging during masturbation is simply pleasure.

Edging is a way to explore your body and make masturbation even more enjoyable. Those who edge report not only enjoying the experience of waxing and waning arousal and riding the orgasmic line, but experiencing more intense orgasms when they do allow themselves to climax. These edging sessions may last ten to twenty minutes or three to four hours, depending on how well someone can block out their afternoon schedule.

For those who are on the extreme edge of edging, these marathon sessions can result in *gooning*. Although gooning stems from the word *goon*, meaning "stupid person," the term is not used by self-labeled gooners derogatorily. Instead, the term describes losing mental ability during masturbation and entering a trance-like state in which someone feels as if they are one with their penis.

Unsurprisingly, empirical evidence is lacking on the phenomenon of gooning, so we are left with anecdotal reports from gooners themselves describing the practice and the transcendental experience. Michael Stahl of *Mel Magazine* took a deep dive into the world of gooning, exploring its dedicated subreddits and practitioners. As "an almost hypnotic, semi-meditative mental state a person can enter after prolonged masturbation," gooning is described as an advanced form of edging that may take some practice in order to enter "goon space." It is at this point, as one gooner described it, where your "mind merges with your cock."

But gooning isn't the only behavior existing on the margins of masturbation. There is more to self-exploration than merely rubbing the pleasurable spots of the penis and clitoris with your hand or a toy. Once someone learns the basic skills of being able to orgasm and to control the timing of orgasm, masturbation adventurers can explore and try novel techniques on their journey of solo pleasure.

Narcissistic or Just Flexible?

The act of sucking one's own penis (formally known as *auto-fellatio*, and less formally as *self-sucking*) has been depicted in pottery and paintings by envious artists for millennia. However, the first clinical documentation of auto-fellatio didn't appear until 1938, with a publication in the *American Journal of Psychiatry* titled "A Clinical Note on a Self-Fellator." The three-page report details the characteristics of a thirty-three-year-old sex offender referred for psychiatric evaluation during his incarceration. Despite his history of sexual violence against children and animals, the psychiatrists were most intrigued by and devoted the entire paper to the man's compulsion to suck his own penis.

In the 1940s, Dr. Alfred Kinsey reported many men have at least attempted to self-fellate, but due to our upright skeletal structures, he estimated that less than 0.3 percent of men actually have the flexibility (and necessary penile length) to accomplish this feat. Likely due to its rarity, auto-fellatio is a behavior of legend. In the late nineteenth century, the Italian decadent poet Gabriele D'Annunzio was rumored to have surgically removed some of his rib cage in order to suck his own penis. A similar rumor surfaced in the 1990s about musician Marilyn Manson. Although both rumors were unfounded, the hedonistic personas of both men had most people thinking, *I can believe that.*

In 1971, psychiatrist Dr. Frank Orland believed sucking one's own penis was a sign of psychopathology. To him, auto-fellatio wasn't simply a masturbatory behavior that the anatomically fortunate found pleasurable. Instead, it was a symptom of self-centeredness because the act creates a literal "ring of narcissism," like some sort of egotistical ouroboros.

The psychiatry and psychology fields have largely ignored this behavior, aside from a small handful of sensational case reports from the 1930s through the 1970s, in which the authors frame the behavior as a form of sexual deviance and a manifestation of latent homosexuality (also viewed as sexually deviant). This view is common, too, among laypeople who think sucking one's own penis is "gay" and that it would likely feel more like giving a blow job than receiving one. But the reality is that, regardless of sexual orientation, auto-fellatio is simply a pleasurable behavior. Aside from the risk of a sore neck, if you have the anatomical gifts, feel free to indulge in self-sucking as you desire and without worrying about what it says about your identity.

Canals of Pleasure

When I teach a sexual health class to students or psychology interns, I often include a segment on sexual slang terms where I have the attendees attempt to define a particular word. This not only increases everyone's knowledge of various slang about sexual behavior, but also increases their comfort in discussing sexuality, often in explicit and graphic detail.

However, one such term, *muffing*, is typically met with dumbfounded silence, as it is a foreign word for most of my students. Nevertheless, I encourage guesses as to what they think it means, and the answers have ranged from cunnilingus to scissoring to dry-humping a blueberry muffin.

I'm not sure why it had to be blueberry.

Occasionally, a student will be better versed in trans women's sexuality, and will know that muffing means fingering the inguinal canals, a term coined by Mira Bellweather, who wrote the zine *Fucking Trans Women* in 2010. The inguinal canals are the openings inside the body between the scrotum and pelvis, where the vas deferens passes through and where the testes originally descended from during fetal development.

The diameter of the canals is about the size of a finger, which lends itself to the creationist argument that God made the human body to be muffed.

Muffing can stimulate the ilioinguinal and genitofemoral nerves, both of which originate in the lumbar region of the spinal cord and pass through the inguinal canals into the scrotum. For some muffers, stimulating these nerves through the canals can be pleasurable. And while the medical literature on muffing is nonexistent, Dr. Curtis Crane, a Texas plastic surgeon and reconstructive urologist specializing in gender affirmation surgeries, told *Vice* that he has never heard of a "muffing injury."

So despite the novelty and unknown territory of fingering the hole inside your own scrotum, there seems to be very little risk of such a practice. Muff away as you please.

Don't Breathe

While auto-fellatio and muffing carry very little risk for an adventurous masturbator to explore, a much more common masturbatory behavior, autoerotic asphyxiation, carries considerable risk if not practiced cautiously. Autoerotic asphyxiation involves limiting, restricting, or obstructing breathing capabilities or blood flow to the brain during masturbation. While similar in function and arousal to choking during partnered sex, autoerotic asphyxiation relies on the use of ligatures (e.g., belts, ropes), masks, or other devices that can be self-administered.

In a 2019 study of 395 Canadians recruited on social media (and subreddits for BDSM), a third of the participants were very or somewhat repulsed by autoerotic asphyxiation, but 42 percent reported mild to strong sexual arousal when engaging in the behavior. Of those who practice it, over 80 percent were not distressed by the behavior, and it correlated with general masochistic interest. It typically develops in late adolescence and is discovered through reading about it online (but only 16 percent learned about it from porn).

Of particular concern, 19 percent of the participants in the study who engaged in autoerotic asphyxiation did not use any safety precautions to protect against accidental death. This is concerning because a review of the literature from 1954 to 2004 found fifty-seven forensic pathology articles detailing 408 cases of accidental death from autoerotic asphyxiation. Practitioners, who were mainly white males between the ages of nine and seventy-seven, typically died from hanging or another form of ligature, but 10.3 percent of deaths were caused by associated accidents through electrocution or foreign body insertion while the person was suffocating themselves.

The reason this masturbatory behavior has gotten so much academic, clinical, and forensic attention is that it is difficult for first responders, investigators, and medical examiners to determine whether the death was accidental or intentional via suicide or homicide. During my undergraduate years, I took a criminal justice course called Equivocal Death Investigation, in which we read pathology reports, examined crime scene photos, and watched home movies made by people who have died during this practice. It became apparent that the accidental deaths were typically caused by not rigging the ligatures to release should the person start losing consciousness. For the deceased, the ropes only became tighter as their body went limp. Watching a video of a man masturbating while accidentally and slowly hanging himself to death was not the college experience my high school guidance counselor promised me.

An X–Rated Mind's Eye

On a lighter note, knowing thyself is not limited to simply knowing your anatomy and what kind of touch turns you on. It is also knowing the desired erotic world you can create through fantasy that increases and facilitates the pleasure of masturbation. Dr. Justin Lehmiller, a social psychologist and research fellow at the Kinsey Institute, studied fantasies among a non-representative sample of over four thousand Americans. Much like the seemingly impossible sexual feat of auto-fellatio, a surprising 20 percent of women and 10 percent of men reported experiencing an orgasm from sexual fantasy alone, without any self-rubbing of penises or clitorises.

But for most people unable to perform this hands-free parlor trick, fantasy is merely a supplement to physical masturbation. In Dr. Lehmiller's study, later published in his book *Tell Me What You Want*, seven fantasy themes emerged as the most common:

1. Sex with multiple partners—Most commonly threesomes, but also includes group sex, gangbangs, and orgies.
2. Power exchange—Anything that involves BDSM (bondage, discipline/dominance, submission/sadism, masochism). This includes both consensual and non-consensual scenarios (about half of the men and two-thirds of the women in the study reported rape fantasies).
3. Novelty and variety—Fantasies that deviate from the Friday night routine, including trying new behaviors (e.g., anal sex), new positions (e.g., reverse cowgirl), or new settings (e.g., sex in parks or confessional booths).

4. Taboo or forbidden—Around 60 percent of the study's sample reported fantasizing about watching other people have sex, also known as voyeurism. Fewer than half (42 percent) fantasized about showing their genitals to a willing partner, whereas 10 percent had exhibitionistic fantasies involving an unsuspecting stranger.

5. Non-monogamy—This fantasy includes partner swap and swinging, but one of the most common non-monogamy fantasies is cuckolding, with 58 percent of the men in the study reporting they masturbate to the thought of their girlfriend or wife having sex with another man.

6. Intimacy and romance—Not all fantasies involve dressing up like Dracula and having sex with the other moms in the PTA. Some fantasies focus less on the sexual behaviors, and more on the feelings of being desired and validated.

7. Homoeroticism and gender bending—For straight and cisgender survey participants, common fantasies emerged about having sex with those of the same gender and cross-dressing.

It is important to note that these seven themes are not mutually exclusive categories. For example, a straight man with a cuckolding fantasy that involves watching his wife have sex with another guy, forced to suck on the man's penis, and all three snuggling afterwards, is an example of a very specific fantasy that incorporates all seven themes.

Also of note, a question I regularly get asked from anxious fantasizers is how common their particular fantasy is. I understand the motivation behind such a question; they are just looking for some validation and to be told they are normal. However, in my opinion, percentages reflecting the prevalence or normalcy of fantasies are meaningless. You can be the only one with a particular fantasy and it be perfectly healthy. If you fantasize about having sex with the Rice Krispies elves while your former kindergarten teacher watches, there's nothing inherently unhealthy or wrong about that, despite its likely low prevalence. And given the fact that I was able to quickly come up with that unlikely scenario, I'm probably not the first one to think of it. If you can think of it, it's probably been done, and someone has probably made a genre of porn about it.

The concern over the normalcy of fantasies is also rooted in concerns about acting on those fantasies, especially if the fantasy involves unethical or illegal behavior or if that fantasy goes against your sexual values. But fantasies do not have to be acted upon. Fantasies aren't necessarily urges. There are a host of reasons why a fantasy would only stay in the head of a masturbator, including health and safety concerns, the legality or ethics of acting on the fantasy, or simply the logistics of trying to coordinate the schedules of twenty-nine furries for a gangbang.

Instead of worrying about where a fantasy is originating from, if it's normal, if it's healthy, if it's socially acceptable, or what it means about your sexuality, simply accept the fantasy for what it is: a fleeting thought that is sexually arousing that is helping you masturbate.

It doesn't have to be anything more than that.

This is your erotic world that you are creating for yourself. You are the ruler over your own body; do with it as you please. There is literally nothing that can come between you and a self-induced orgasm. That is, of course, unless you want to buy a dildo in Texas.

CHAPTER 7

Dildo Control

Vibrators, Sex Dolls, and Foreign Body Insertions

Dawn Webber was in Austin, Texas, in early 2000, working her managerial shift at the aptly named Adult Video Store when Lori Carlin walked in looking to buy a dildo. Webber assisted Carlin by showing her various options and educating her about the stimulating features of each. Carlin selected a dildo of interest and proceeded to purchase it at the cash register. What Webber didn't know at the time was that Carlin was an undercover cop working for the Travis County Sheriff's Department.

Once the purchase was made, Webber was arrested by Deputy Sheriff Charles Jones who was monitoring the dildo sting operation via live video. In transit to the sheriff's department, Webber allegedly told the deputies, "I've been arrested for selling this before and I'll go to jail for it again." She was subsequently charged with violating Texas Penal Code 43.21 and 43.23, which prohibits the selling of "any obscene material or device . . . including a dildo or artificial vagina, designed and marketed as useful primarily for stimulation of the human genital organs."

During the trial, Deputy Carlin testified about the purchased device, saying there was no "mistaking the shape of this dildo for anything other than a male penis" and that it was to be used solely for sexual gratification. During cross-examination, Webber's defense attorney unsuccessfully argued that the dildo wasn't inherently made for masturbation, and that the device could be purchased and used as a paperweight or a doorstop. Jurors weren't convinced, and they found Webber guilty of the abominable crime of selling a non-paperweight dildo to a cop.

The morally zealous prosecutor sought a one-year prison sentence for Webber to protect the public from having orgasms. The court ultimately decided on a sentence of thirty days in the county jail and a fine of $4,000.

Thirty days in jail for selling a dildo in America.

Webber also lost her appeal to have the ruling overturned, but a reluctantly concurring judge did note the ridiculousness of the law and its discretionary enforcement. Every jurisdiction has archaic laws that have never been officially invalidated,[39] but the Travis County Sheriff's Department made the conscious decision to devote at least two deputies to investigate and arrest a woman selling a dildo. Instead of mocking the arresting officers and telling them to focus on gun violence prevention or literally anything else, the Travis County prosecutor proceeded to indict Webber, convince a jury that she's a moral danger to the state, and seek the maximum penalty for her offense to Texas decency.

Treating the selling of dildos as more dangerous to the general public than the selling of handguns and semiautomatic rifles is not uniquely Texan. The state governments of Louisiana, Mississippi, and Alabama share similar values with the governments of Saudi Arabia, Malaysia, and the United Arab Emirates, all of whom also share a commitment to restricting abortion access, prohibiting comprehensive sex education, and protecting the public from the corrupting influence of a vibrating penis and a silicone vagina.

---

39. It is a felony in Michigan for a man to "seduce or debauch any unmarried woman." In Nebraska, seventeen-year-olds can get married as long as they don't have gonorrhea.

Fortunately for Texans, though, two sex toy companies filed a law-suit against the state in 2007. The companies argued that the law pro-hibiting the sale of "obscene devices" violated Texans' right to privacy protected under the Fourteenth Amendment of the US Constitution.

The state's attorney general (and later Texas governor) Greg Abbott decided it was a good use of everyone's time and state resources to defend the overreaching and unnecessary law. As solicitor general working under Attorney General Abbott, current US Senator Ted Cruz argued, "There is no substantive due-process right to stimulate one's genitals for non-medical reasons unrelated to procreation or outside of an interper-sonal relationship." This was part of his coauthored eighty-three-page legal brief arguing on behalf of the state of Texas why criminalizing dildo selling was necessary in "protecting public morals" and that the govern-ment should have a commitment to discouraging "autonomous sex."

The legal brief also argued that the law does not violate the privacy rights of Texans because it does not target the "obscene device user" (i.e., the masturbator), but criminalizes the sale of these devices deemed obscene.[40] Additionally, Solicitor General Cruz argued that legalizing the sale of dildos for sexual gratification would be a slippery slope to decriminalizing sex work.

Ultimately, the plaintiffs won their lawsuit and Texans are able to freely sell sex toys and own more than five vibrators without fear of get-ting arrested by the dildo police.

A Brief History of Sex Toys

Much like attitudes toward masturbation, the legalization and utiliza-tion of sex toys have not followed a linear progression. One of the oldest

---

40. However, owning six or more sex toys is a crime. The state of Texas views ownership of this many dildos as evidence of intent to sell. Unrelated, there is no law capping the number of firearms a person can own in the Lone Star State.

dildos ever discovered was found at an archaeological dig site in southern Germany in 2005.[41] At nearly eight inches long, the siltstone object was sculpted 28,000 years ago and polished to resemble a human penis, but there is debate over its use and function among the Ice Age European inhabitants. There is physical evidence to suggest it was used as a sharpening tool for flint arrowheads, but given the fact that a sharpening tool does not have to be molded into the shape of a penis to be functional, there is speculation that it may have also been symbolic art, incorporated into rituals, or used on the genitals for sexual stimulation.

Likewise, dildos (or artistic representations of dildos) have been discovered in archaeological dig sites all over the world, from Pakistan to China to Egypt, dating from 2,500 to 30,000 years old. Detachable penises are also widely depicted in art and literature from ancient Greece and the Roman Empire. As soon as humans were writing on walls, dildos were being crafted and finding their place within human civilization.

By the seventeenth century, dildos were widespread across Europe and Asia. However, England saw them as a threat to society and confiscated (and dramatically burned) any dildo that was imported. While the English saw dildos as an insult to men and masculinity, the Japanese embraced them as playful and harmless toys. Throughout the seventeenth century in Japan, depictions of sex toys commonly appeared in erotic books as a pleasurable device for women. But, ultimately, both the erotica and sex toys were banned from Japan beginning in 1722.

Vibrators, on the other hand, the most commonly used sex toy today, have a much more recent history. It is often believed that vibrators were invented (or at least widely used) as a medical device to cure

---

41. The dildo was found in the Hohle Fels cave where the famous nude Venus figurine was also discovered, which is the first example of figurative art by humans. Although not inherently sexual, I'm sure there was at least one Paleolithic German who masturbated while gazing upon the figurine's bosom.

women's hysteria in the eighteenth century. Hysteria, of course, being clinically defined as a woman expressing any emotion that makes a man uncomfortable. As lovely as the thought of a doctor from 1870 cranking up a rickety electric vibrator to soothe the hysterics of a woman may be, this story is nothing more than an urban legend.

Although written as science-fiction horror in 1818, Mary Shelley's *Frankenstein* offered a glimpse of the marvels of electricity and what curative powers may lie ahead. Residents of Victorian England had an obsession with electricity. The newly developed electric vibrator, first patented by English physician Joseph Mortimer Granville in the 1880s, was originally designed to help alleviate muscle aches in men, not women. And although the vibrator was later marketed as a tool to cure a whole host of ills, including headaches, constipation, and cancer, vibrators were not being used on clitorises by doctors to cure "hysterical women."[42]

By 1915, the American Medical Association argued that the claims about the curative power of vibration were unfounded, and if there were any effects, they were placebo effects. As a result, vibrators moved away from being marketed as medical devices and toward being marketed as domestic appliances much like "personal massagers" are today.

Even though vibrators were not being directly marketed for masturbation, Dr. Hallie Lieberman, author of *Buzz: A Stimulating History of the Sex Toy*, speculates that home vibrators were being used for masturbation by the early twentieth century. It often doesn't take long

---

42. The myth is largely attributed to claims made in the 1999 book *The Technology of Orgasm* by historian Dr. Rachel Maines. The book has been widely cited by academics, which only strengthened the urban legend and inspired documentaries, a Broadway play, and the movie *Hysteria*, starring Maggie Gyllenhaal. When confronted by other historians about the accuracy and documented support for her claim that vibrators were invented to treat hysteria in women, Dr. Maines defensively argued that they were "just theories," which is academic jargon for "I made it up."

for people to create makeshift vibrators from existing appliances, like sewing machines. Sex historian Dr. Kate Lister refers to this as the *kink blink*—the short amount of time it takes for someone to utilize a new invention in a masturbatory manner. Used in a sentence, "The 1990s' fad squiggle pen went from a fun way to write in your diary to someone's first clitoral vibrator in a kink blink."

In the 1970s, sex-positive feminists like Betty Dodson viewed vibrators not only as a tool for self-discovery and orgasmic pleasure, but also for sexual revolution and liberation. As the vibrator moved out of the domestic appliance realm and began being advertised in home goods catalogs, it moved into the public sphere through lectures, workshops, and feminist-owned stores like Good Vibrations in San Francisco.[43] As an extension of "the personal is political," masturbating with a vibrator became an act of resistance to heteronormativity and patriarchal phallocentrism that often minimized, if not completely disregarded, female pleasure and orgasm.

Possibly to the chagrin of the sexual radicals of the 1970s, the focus on using vibrators became less about collective political resistance in the form of gender and sexual liberation at the close of the twentieth century, but more about neoliberal, individual empowerment in the form of self-help consumer choices. It lost its appeal as a device for revolution and became a toy for recreational pleasure.

Mainstream consumer demand for vibrators meant manufacturers and retailers began offering vibrators to meet the functional and aesthetic needs of every conceivable masturbator. Vibrators are now offered in a variety of colors and range in size from as small as a pinkie finger to

---

43. Joani Blank, the founder of Good Vibrations, established National Masturbation Day on May 7, 1995, in honor of Dr. Jocelyn Elders. The day has since been expanded to the entire month of May being known as National Masturbation Month. Plan your early summer adventures accordingly.

as large as a forearm. Shapes vary, too, and may resemble penises, tubes of lipstick, roses, electric toothbrushes, and ergonomically designed computer mice.

The new millennium also saw the mainstreaming of vibrators when they became commonplace in movies, television shows, retail stores, and even Tupperware-like at-home parties. Arguably one of the most influential pop culture references was in an episode of HBO's *Sex and the City*. Already known for its frank discussions of sexual behavior, the first season's ninth episode depicted Charlotte, the more conservative woman in the group, purchasing a vibrator known as the Rabbit. Relieved that the experience of buying a vibrator in a sex shop was less intimidating than expected, she excitedly exclaimed, "Oh, it's so cute! I thought it would be scary and weird, but it isn't. It's pink! For girls!"

Characteristics of the Obscene Device User

Charlotte's excitement over her new purchase (that ultimately had her friends staging an intervention over her "Rabbit habit") ushered in a new era of vibrator consumerism. Sex shop retailers like Carol Queen of Good Vibrations in San Francisco and Jacq Jones of Sugar in Baltimore recalled sales of vibrators spiking for years after the airing of the *Sex and the City* episode, with many women asking for the Rabbit by name. The episode normalized buying and using vibrators that undoubtedly increased demand for quality sex toys.

Examining the characteristics of vibrator users, Dr. Debby Herbenick, a public health professor at Indiana University's Center for Sexual Health Promotion, published a series of studies between 2009 and 2017. Dr. Herbenick found that 51.2 percent of women and 38.2 percent of men reported that using a vibrator is at least somewhat appealing. A similar percentage of women and men have used a vibrator at least once in their lifetime, and 20 percent of women and 5.5 percent of men reported a vibration adventure in the past month.

And those 20 percent of women may have the upper hand sexually. Women who have used a vibrator in the past thirty days are more likely to have better sexual functioning as measured by the Female Sexual Functioning Index, a nineteen-item questionnaire developed at the Robert Wood Johnson Medical School's Department of Psychiatry that assesses difficulties with sexual desire, arousal, orgasm, and pain. Furthermore, vibrator use among women is associated with those who have gotten a gynecological exam in the past year and have closely examined their own genitals in the past month, which are two behaviors that are correlated with better sexual health.

Less is known about the motivations, barriers, and experiences of using vibrators from interview-based studies, but two researchers— Dr. Dennis Waskul, a sociology professor at Minnesota State University, Mankato, and social worker Michelle Anklan—tried to fill this knowledge gap with the publication of their 2020 academic article, "'Best Invention, Second to the Dishwasher': Vibrators and Sexual Pleasure."

For the participants in this study, it was common to first learn about vibrators between the ages of twelve and fourteen from social media, movies, friends, and family. Unlike the many social learning myths surrounding porn use and influencing sexual development, only 4.7 percent of the participants first became aware of vibrators from watching porn.

But within mainstream movies and television shows like *Sex and the City*, the participants felt there was a contradiction in how vibrator use was represented. On the one hand, vibrators were portrayed as a fun and pleasurable device, and a way to have agency and autonomy over one's own sex life. On the other hand, participants felt that vibrators were also portrayed as a "dirty secret." And for one participant who didn't mince words, she felt the media portrayed vibrators like nothing more than a "dick substitute."

Many participants felt unsure as to how to use a vibrator or how their body would respond, which the authors speculated was due to our cultural ignorance about anatomy and physiology. Although many participants felt that using a vibrator felt "foreign and unnatural" at first, these worries were quickly abated through experimentation and trial and error. Once learning how their body responded, 76.14 percent believed vibrator use changed their capacity to achieve orgasm for the better. One participant commented, "Before, I would masturbate by watching porn and using my fingers. With a vibrator, I don't have to watch porn to be able to orgasm." This anecdote about not watching porn should be good news for groups like Fight the New Drug. But, then again, I'm sure the organization would launch a new campaign to fight the *new* new drug—vibrators.

Vibrator Addiction

Concerns about clitoral desensitization from vibrator use is a common question I have received from students and patients over the past decade. The fear is likely rooted in uncertainty and insecurity over masturbating in general, and with sex toys specifically, but also a cultural value of prioritizing pleasure derived from partnered sex as the most important sexual behavior. This belief serves as a barrier for women's willingness to use vibrators and has their sexual partners expressing insecurity that they'll be replaced by something with batteries.

Of the participants interviewed and surveyed in Dr. Waskul's study, almost 18 percent were worried they would become dependent on their vibrator or that it would decrease the pleasure during partnered sexual activity. Masters and Johnson were concerned about this in the 1970s, speculating that a woman could become desensitized and dependent on vibrators to the point of no longer being able to have an orgasm through partnered intercourse.

Fortunately, clitoral desensitization from vibrator use is an unfounded fear and myth. Dr. Clive Davis, an associate professor emeritus of psychology at Syracuse University, researched this fear in 1996 and found that most of the women in his sample reported more intense orgasms with a vibrator than without, and less than 10 percent reported only being able to orgasm from a vibrator. However, even among the 10 percent of women in this study who relied on a vibrator to reach orgasm, the inability to orgasm without a vibrator was not caused by repeated vibrator use. For these women, a vibrator was the only thing that had ever allowed them to orgasm.

In short, the clitoris does not lose its ability to pleasurably respond to stimulation from using a vibrator, despite what your insecure boyfriend tries to tell you.

However, what can happen is that vibrators can provide an avenue to orgasm that is highly pleasurable and efficient, and your body may become conditioned to responding to this very specific type of touch. This does not mean the clitoris is desensitized or that you have developed a dependence on sex toys. You just found the most efficient and enjoyable way to reach an orgasm. This can happen with penile masturbation, too (sometimes referred to as idiosyncratic masturbation or "death grip syndrome"), where someone's masturbation technique is an exciting and efficient way to reach orgasm alone, but the technique doesn't replicate well with a partner.

When this situation is brought up in therapy, the goal is not to take away the pleasure from masturbation, but to add more pleasure to partnered sex. You found a way that works amazingly for you alone; now you just need to find a way that also works for you with a partner. And this is where the knowledge about your sexual response from masturbation is useful information. You may need more direct stimulation on your clitoris during sex, which is currently lacking in order to reach orgasm, and that might include using a vibrator during sex.

The vibrator is not an enemy of or a competitor to a partner. It can be an ally, a teammate, and a friend. Therefore, just as it's an important reminder to replace the batteries in your vibrator, it's important to replace your boyfriend if they are intimidated by your vibrator.

The German Spot

With the marketing of vibrators as personal devices for sexual empowerment, some sex toys make large promises to bring the user to heightened states of ecstasy never experienced before. Some make this promise by marketing sex toys as a "g-spot stimulator," and for only $59.99, mind-blowing orgasms and large gushes of ejaculation await.

In 1950, the German gynecologist Ernst Gräfenberg first described a potential erogenous zone on the front wall of the vagina. Published in the *International Journal of Sexology*, Dr. Gräfenberg's article, "The Role of the Urethra in Female Orgasm," reported that the area surrounding a woman's urethra consists of erectile tissue similar to the structure of the penis, and that this area enlarges during sexual stimulation.

In 1981, Dr. Beverly Whipple and colleagues published "Female Ejaculation: A Case Study" in the *Journal of Sex Research*, describing this erogenous zone as a specific spot and naming it, after its founder, the *Gräfenberg spot* (or g-spot for those who can't pronounce German). The idea of a hidden "pleasure button" became mainstream and popularized a year later with the publication of Dr. Whipple's bestselling book *The G-Spot and Other Recent Discoveries about Human Sexuality*.

The book was an instant hit and was a rare occurrence of women's sexual pleasure getting attention and being valued. All of a sudden, women were searching for this legendary spot with fingers and toys with the promise of mind-blowing orgasms.

However, not all women were able to successfully locate their g-spot. Even after buying sex toys specifically designed and marketed to be able to stimulate the spot, some women felt shortchanged if they felt nothing special when that area of the vaginal wall was stimulated. This prompted some in the sexual health field to criticize the book's conclusions, arguing that anecdotes or studies with small samples were not sufficient to make bold claims about a universal pleasure spot.

Also, considering that studies involving dissected cadavers have found no unique anatomical structure that could be labeled the g-spot, there has been a more recent effort to move away from thinking there is a unique and specific *spot* along the front wall of the vagina. Instead, to take the pressure off finding a specific spot, think of the area as a potential erogenous *zone*. This zone is part of the cliterourethral-vaginal complex.[44]

Gushers

To add more unnecessary mystery to female sexual anatomy and functioning, controversy not only surrounds the naming of sensitive vaginal tissue as a spot or a zone, but, for some women, there is the experience of ejaculating some type of fluid during sexual stimulation, with 10 to 54 percent of women reporting they have expelled fluid during arousal or orgasm.

The debate over female ejaculation (or squirting) is whether the fluid is similar to semen, vaginal lubrication, or urine. The most recent review of the literature from 2017 suggests it could be all three.

---

44. For the sake of spellcheck, please someone in the medical field officially shorten that to the CUV complex.

Clitoris Tourist

In Anatomy 101, the external part of the clitoris, known as the glans clitoris, is just the tip of the iceberg. Most of the clitoris is internal, with the shaft extending inward from the glans, and then branching off into sets of bulbs and legs (called crura if you want to sound fancy). This internal structure surrounds the urethra and the vagina, thus allowing indirect stimulation of the clitoris from inserting a finger, vibrator, or dildo into the vagina.

Freud argued that there is a difference between clitoral and vaginal orgasms, and stated that clitoral orgasms are "immature" because they reflect an early psychosexual stage of development involving "penis envy," whereas a vaginal orgasm demonstrates developmental maturity because the woman is having an orgasm involving her reproductive tract. The reality is, physiologically, there is no difference between clitoral and vaginal orgasms. Although there may be different subjective feelings about experiencing an orgasm from stimulating different body parts, physiologically, an orgasm is an orgasm. This is because the cliterourethralvaginal complex is a network of nerves, erectile tissue, and glands that are activated with any kind of genital stimulation, whether it's external or internal.

Using a vibrator just on your glans clitoris? The cliterourethralvaginal complex is being stimulated.

Using a specially designed g-spot vibrator on the front wall of your vagina? The cliterourethralvaginal complex is being stimulated.

Therefore, if your vibrator feels the best externally, it doesn't mean you are missing out on finding a spot internally. And vice versa. Simply ask yourself, "Does it feel good?" If yes, great. Keep pleasuring yourself exactly where it is most satisfying. You do not need a dissected cadaver to validate or invalidate your pleasure.

Vaginal lubrication is an ultra-filtrate of blood plasma that results from increased blood flow during sexual arousal. It is secreted from the walls of the vagina (think of the vagina "sweating" during arousal), and may also contain fluid from the uterus, cervix, and the Bartholin's glands (two small glands located on the lower portion on each side of the vaginal opening, which are homologous to the Cowper's glands in men that secrete "pre-cum"). It has high potassium and low sodium concentrations. For some women, a small amount of fluid may be expelled through the vaginal opening during orgasm from muscular contractions of the vagina.

Female ejaculation, in contrast to vaginal lubrication, is a thick, milky fluid expelled from the urethral opening. Usually a tablespoon or less, the fluid is believed to originate from the Skene's glands, which is tissue homologous to the prostate. Similar to prostate fluid in semen, female ejaculate contains high concentrations of prostate-specific antigen (PSA), glucose, phosphatase, and fructose. The ducts of the gland enter into the urethra and expel fluid through the urethral opening. Researchers are not quite sure of the function of this fluid (it may be comparable to useless male nipples), but it also may have antimicrobial properties to protect the urinary tract from infection. Regardless, this information makes a great conversation starter at family reunions.

Lastly, squirting (or gushing) is a term that is often used synonymously with female ejaculation, but it is different from ejaculate and vaginal lubrication in terms of its color, consistency, and volume; it is clear, watery, and the expulsion can range from 15 to 110 milliliters.[45] Also, since the fluid originates from the bladder and is expelled through

---

45. For Americans unable to conceptualize metric volume, squirting fluid can range from a tablespoon to a little more than what you're allowed to bring on an airplane in a single container.

the urethral opening, it has a chemical composition of diluted urine or a composition exactly similar to urine.

So is the fluid expelled during masturbation, often at orgasm, pee? Maybe, sometimes. It depends on what the fluid looks like, the amount, and the opening it's coming from. If it's clear, watery, and coming out of the urethral opening in a large amount, then the fluid is likely coming from the bladder and is indistinguishable from diluted urine.

But does that matter?

Dr. Jessica Påfs, a senior lecturer and researcher at the University of Gothenburg, studied Swedish women's experience with squirting and ejaculation to better understand the importance placed on this phenomenon. Many of the interviewees felt amazed by their body's ability to ejaculate and felt as if it opened a new part of their sexuality. They felt part of the sexual elite, with several women who referred to it as a "sexual superpower" and a feminist ability, saying, "I am fascinated about it and I think it feels like such an amazing power and a feminist statement, almost like throwing it back in their face, you might say, after all these years of oppression of women's sexuality."

Some of the women reported greater pleasure from it, like an emptying sensation, but not everyone felt it gave them more physical pleasure at orgasm. Others felt let down because there was not much fluid expelled and/or there wasn't greater sensation with orgasm, as if it wasn't living up to its hype. Several of the women were discomforted by the wetness and mess it created with sex, as well as being uncomfortable with squirting being associated with promiscuity, hypersexuality, and pornography. And a few women had partners who were disgusted at the sight of the fluid or its expulsion, resulting in shame and embarrassment for the squirter or ejaculator.

Questions and insecurity about fluid expulsion have arisen in therapy and the classroom throughout my career, reflecting the reports based on Dr. Påfs's research. While it is understandable to fall prey to our culture's negative messaging around female orgasms, it is important to focus on owning your bodily responses and the pleasure that comes from them. Regardless of what the fluid is or where it comes from, if it feels good expelling it during masturbation, embrace it.

Culturally, we have no problem with semen going wherever it wants to, and have viewed its expulsion as not only a normal and healthy part of sexual behavior, but as an indicator that sexual behavior has taken place and is completed. There is comical acceptance of stained sheets and crusty tube socks. Even if it means you need to invest in a few more bath towels, give your fluid the same ejaculatory freedom as semen. As grind-gore metal band Brutal Sphincter once screamed in their un-rhyming song "The Art of Squirting," "Squealing in pleasure is the ultimate goal you'll achieve, aim for the wall and make some modern art!"

Prostate Milking

Much like the shape and function of g-spot vibrators to stimulate ejaculation, there are specific sex toys designed for anal insertion to stimulate the prostate gland through the rectal wall in the hopes of orgasm and ejaculation. Often referred to as the p-spot or the male g-spot,[46] the prostate can be a hidden gem of self-induced pleasure. With a lack of NIH research grants to study butt play, most of the research on prostate-induced orgasms is anecdotal, with men reporting more intense orgasms than from penile stimulation alone, often referring to them as "Super-Os." While it may take more time, effort, and skill to pleasurably stimulate the prostate, butt self-explorers have anecdotally reported that

---

46. I find amusing the unnecessarily gendered language of g-spots and prostates. G-spots can produce female ejaculation, whereas male g-spots can produce ejaculation. This would be like calling the clitoris the female penis, and calling the ovaries the male testicles.

prostate orgasms can culminate in twelve pelvic muscle contractions, compared to the measly four to eight contractions from penile orgasms.

As with g-spot stimulation and squirting, taboos and insecurities surround men anally masturbating to stimulate their prostate. Among the biggest insecurities is the stereotypical association between anal eroticism and homosexuality, which prompts straight men to shy away from their buttholes.

But despite what homophobic televangelists may think, the anus does not have a sexual orientation. Ask any proctologist,[47] and they will tell you there is no anatomical or neurological difference in the anuses, rectums, and prostates between gay and straight men. Pleasure is pleasure. Engaging in prostate self-stimulation does not mean you are secretly desiring to have anal sex with a man any more than masturbating by hand means you are desiring to get a hand job by your buddy Frank.

But with anal insertion of sex toys, on the quest to stimulate the prostate, comes great responsibility to avoid autoerotic mishaps.

Don't Be a Case Study

As my grandma used to say, "Anything's a dildo if you're brave enough."[48] For the vast majority of sex toy users (even those brave enough to try unique household items as sexual stimulants), the outcome of masturbating with an object is going to simply be self-pleasure, not self-harm. But for the unlucky few, what started out as an adventure in penetrative pleasure turned into a trip to the emergency room.

---

47. This is a rhetorical statement. Don't waste a proctologist's time asking them this silly question.

48. My grandma likely never said that. The origin of the phrase dates back to an anonymous social media user in 2011 who used it as a "troll quote," attributing the phrase to US President Abraham Lincoln. It has since become a meme and is often attached to photos of large, phallic-shaped objects.

As was the case in 1919, when Dr. Orvall Smiley published a case report in the *Journal of the American Medical Association*, titled "A Glass Tumbler in the Rectum." The report notes that a fifty-five-year-old man from Indiana brought himself to the hospital after anally inserting a glass tumbler for sexual pleasure *two days* earlier. Unable to remove the tumbler back through the anus, the surgeon cut open the man's abdominal cavity and large intestine to remove the slightly broken, 3-by-4-inch tumbler. Although the extraction was a success, the short, three-paragraph case report abruptly concludes with the morbid sentence, "The patient died sixteen hours later."

When it comes to anal insertion of objects for masturbation, men outnumber women thirty-seven to one. Maybe it is the novelty or the taboo or attempts to stimulate the prostate, but men love putting things in their butts. One ER physician in 2022 reported removing twenty Happy Meal toys from a middle-aged man's anus, which gives a new meaning to the McDonald's slogan, "I'm lovin' it."

Medical case reports have been written about many men's pursuits of self-pleasure via foreign body insertion into the anus. Cases detail a plethora of inserted objects, including glasses, silverware, hangers, and most household items. Pretty much everything that was on your sister's wedding registry has been in a man's rectum.

Unfortunately, though, death by prostate pilgrimaging did not die in 1919. Other case reports from 2007 and 2021 detail fatal masturbatory adventures in articles titled "Vibrator-Induced Fatal Rectal Perforation" and "Rectal Explosion: A Strange Case of Autoerotic Death." And although these cases were the result of two men having eyes bigger than their rectums, masturbatory injuries from butt exploration have prompted sex toy companies to design vibrators, dildos, and butt plugs with safety in mind by equipping them with flared bases or pull strings to ensure that nothing gets lost inside the colon in pursuit of pleasure.

But, butts aren't the only orifice masturbators may explore and ultimately find themselves the subjects of a physician's case study. The insertion of foreign bodies is known as the nearly unpronounceable clinical term, *polyembolokoilamania*. This includes insertion of objects into any bodily orifice, including the anus, vagina, urethra, mouth, nose, and ears. Vaginal injuries have been reported from prolonged insertion of household objects and sports equipment like tennis balls, leading to infection with septic shock and air entering the bloodstream. Although the motivations for foreign body insertion can range from non-suicidal self-injury to psychotic disorders, a significant portion of "polyembolo-koilamaniacs" do so for sexual gratification during masturbation, often without a thorough understanding of what can be inserted safely.

Most curious for the average masturbator, I'd imagine, is the insertion of objects into the urethral opening. Known as "sounding," masturbatory urethral penetration can be a pleasurable experience for the adventurous and need not require the attention of a urologist. There are, however, the unlucky few who find themselves with cystitis, increased urinary frequency, genital swelling, tearing of the urethral lining, or urinary retention, as detailed in the 2005 published case study "Urinary Retention with Ruptured Fornix Caused by a Maggot." Here, a forty-seven-year-old German man reported an erotic interest in maggots since childhood and had been inserting them into his urethra during masturbation with increasing frequency as he aged. During an unfortunate masturbation adventure, one maggot did not come out during ejaculation and required the assistance of urological surgeons for its retrieval. Fortunately, the man survived the ordeal, but now has to live with the embarrassment of knowing his fetishistic escapade is written about in the academic journal the *Urologist*.

But to somewhat normalize the maggot man, he is certainly not alone in his urethral curiosity, nor was he inventive. This behavior, even involving animals or animal parts, is nothing new. In 1897, Dr. Francis Packard, a Philadelphia physician, published an article in *Annals of Surgery* that detailed 221 cases of foreign body insertion into the male urethra that were surgically removed from the bladder. Among the discovered objects used for masturbation were lead pencils, cigarette holders, feathers, chalk, toothpicks, leather shoestring, candle wax, and bone crochet needles. And over the past hundred years, physicians have written case studies on medical mishaps of urethral sounding, involving fishing hooks, a coyote's rib, glass stirrers, and a 45-cm-long decapitated snake.

Again, the vast majority of people who masturbate with the aid of objects inserted into the body do so without needing to call 911. It can be done safely. However, the risk of an emergency can be reduced by using objects with a flared base or attached with a string, sterilizing all inserted objects, using lubricant that is compatible with both your body and the object, and avoiding objects with sharp edges and those with the potential to break or explode. Masturbate safely, as no one wants to find themselves the subject of a medical case study.

Masturbate Smarter, Not Harder

Our human ancestors 28,000 years ago spent hours, if not days, laboring over a piece of siltstone carving it into a dildo. However, in the twenty-first century, modern masturbatory technology, including "teledildonics," can now efficiently and often effortlessly aid in the facilitation of self-induced orgasms. There are vibrators that can be synced to your favorite Spotify playlists to pulsate to the beat of your favorite songs. This allows a person the option of having a relaxing evening with the slow vibes of Adele or a near-clit-numbing experience with Slayer.

If someone loves using a masturbation sleeve to stroke their penis, but has ever thought, *I wish I didn't have to physically move my hand up and down while doing this*, now there are devices that plug into an outlet and will stroke your penis for you at the push of a button. The user is able to adjust the device for speed and length of each stroke, and if they're very trusting, someone else can control those settings remotely via an app on their phone.

Furthermore, long gone are the days of unrealistic inflatable dolls used primarily as a gag gift at bachelor parties. The replacement, a new multimillion-dollar industry, is the use of highly realistic silicone sex dolls that are designed to look and feel like real human skin. Unlike masturbation devices like Fleshlights, which are handheld masturbators modeled to resemble a vulva, anus, or mouth, modern sex dolls are complete, human-sized models with limbs, torsos, and heads. Dolls are often created after the likeness of some of the world's most recognizable porn performers, such as Jessica Drake, Asa Akira, and Stormy Daniels. With enough disposable income (dolls can range in price from $3,999 to $7,200), the modern masturbator is able to live out their real fantasies with fake humans.

There is speculation about whether guys who masturbate via sex dolls are merely creative in seeking autonomous sexual outlets or are sex offenders in the making. Arguments supporting the contention that sex doll users are threats to their communities hold that sex dolls promote the objectification of women and the sexual entitlement of men, both of which are implicit characteristics associated with sexual violence. The opposing arguments suggest that sex dolls simply provide a safe sexual outlet for guys looking to masturbate while simulating sex as closely as possible.

A psychological research team in England sought to provide empirical evidence to support one of the assertions about the risks (or lack thereof) of masturbating with a sex doll. Comparing 158 sex doll owners with 135 non-owners, the researchers found that doll owners tended to be older and single compared to non-owners. And despite doll owners having some traits that are associated with sexual violence, like viewing women as unknowable and the world as dangerous, they actually had *lower* levels of sexual aggression proclivity (measured by arousal to and interest in sexual assault scenarios) than non-doll owners.

The obvious motivation to own a sex doll is masturbation, with 70 percent of respondents from a small survey indicating that sexual gratification was the primary motivation to purchase a doll. However, other motivations include emotional intimacy and companionship. Given that doll owners tend to be older, single, and also have lower sexual self-esteem, this may point to some deficits in having sexual relations with women, but it does not point to using the dolls for sexual assault rehearsals.

Although the concern about sex dolls is extreme, it does reflect the moral panic and misinformation surrounding all sex toys and their users. Whether outright criminalized or dismissed as a poor "dick substitute," sex toys are viewed in our culture as a shameful device for a shameful practice. But much like our brains, which evolved to give us the ability to fantasize, we also evolved to be able to use tools. That demonstration of phenomenal brainpower is something our culture should celebrate, not criminalize or stigmatize. Masturbating to orgasm with the assistance of a battery-powered sex toy or with a replica of your favorite porn performer is one of the few examples of human exceptionalism.

CHAPTER 8

Manual Labor

Peep Shows, Camming, and Communal Cumming

Shortly after the midnight celebratory ball drop in Times Square to ring in 1994, US Attorney Rudy Giuliani was sworn in as New York City's 107th mayor. Giuliani defeated incumbent mayor David Dinkins by promising New Yorkers he was going to improve the quality of life on the city's streets by heavily policing petty nuisance crimes, which he incorrectly believed contributed to more serious violent offenses and decreased property values in neighborhoods. Sitting toward the top of his list of criminal enterprises to wage war against was sex workers, who get paid to masturbate in peep shows.

From paying for sex in the "bawdy houses" in the 1800s to watching sexually explicit films in the "grinder houses" in the 1930s, New York City, and in particular Times Square, has earned its title as a sex capital due to its thriving sex industry. Within this industry exist live peep shows, where sex workers strip and often masturbate in front of paying clientele who are separated from the workers by glass (and who are typically masturbating themselves within their private booths). It is paid mutual masturbation with mutual benefits.

Win-win.

Unless you are Mayor Giuliani, trying to attract Disney and other family-friendly[49] businesses to Times Square.

During his campaign, Mayor Giuliani scapegoated sex workers and their places of employment. He argued that they directly caused public health crises (e.g., the AIDS epidemic) and New York's high crime rate, calling sexually oriented businesses "corrosive institutions" that repel "legitimate businesses." But the claim that peep shows cause crime in the surrounding neighborhood is unfounded by sociological research. And there is no evidence to suggest that masturbation within these venues contributes to sexually transmitted infections within the community. You are not going to get herpes from stepping on a dried semen puddle in your Skechers.

Once he was in office, Mayor Giuliani's moral disapproval of the sex industry masquerading as public health and crime reduction policies was implemented in 1995 with the passage of the Adult Entertainment Ordinance. This zoning ordinance prohibited new sex shops from opening, and made it illegal for current sex shops to expand and be within five hundred feet of residences, schools, or places of worship. In midtown Manhattan, it is impossible to walk fifty feet, let alone five hundred, without passing a combination of apartments, schools, and churches. The ordinance was intentionally designed to shut down the sex industry in Times Square and make room for "legitimate businesses" like Red Lobster and the Bubba Gump Shrimp Company.

Fortunately, professional masturbators relied on one loophole in the new zoning ordinance that allowed some peep shows to stay open. Unlike the New York zoning regulation in 1961 that did not differentiate between sexual and non-sexual businesses, the new zoning ordinance

---

49. "Family-friendly" should refer to universal health care and paid parental leave, not a movie without nipples.

defined a sex shop to be any place of business where at least 40 percent was devoted to adult products, services, or entertainment.

This prompted creativity for peep show owners who rushed to offer a variety of non-adult products and services to fly under the radar of the zoning law's enforcement. Many businesses started selling I ♥ NY coffee mugs and Phantom of the Opera keychains alongside peep show booths and VHS copies of *Up and Cummers 10*.

Law professor Jennifer Cook argued in a 2005 article in *City University of New York Law Review* that this battle between the government and the sex industry in Times Square was not new. From her analysis, this conflict ". . . exists as part of an ongoing ebb and flow between exertions of sexuality and shifting sources of political power, resulting in a tyranny against licentiousness, periods of withdrawal, reorganization, and ultimate resurfacing in compliance with existing legal interpretations."

While some businesses were able to reorganize and resurface in compliance with the new ordinance, the majority of peep shows shuttered permanently. By 1997, Times Square was "cleaned up" enough for Mayor Giuliani's biggest catch to gentrify the neighborhood: Disney.

In April of that year, CEO Michael Eisner unveiled Disney's $34 million renovation to the New Amsterdam Theater on 42nd Street. During the public unveiling ceremony, Eisner talked about his initial reluctance to bring Disney to Times Square given the presence of its sex industry. But Eisner said he spoke with Mayor Giuliani about his concerns over the peep shows and porn theaters, and Mayor Giuliani promised, "Michael, they'll be gone."

Although Mayor Giuliani's term ended in 2001, and he was unable to successfully win any subsequent bid for political office, his moral crusade against New York's sex industry in the 1990s is still felt today. The city is safe from those who get paid to masturbate behind a glass wall, and visitors can enjoy family-friendly and healthy businesses like Olive

Garden and the M&M Candy Store. Tourists from Ohio can safely go to Times Square and find the comforts of their hometown mall without having to worry about the unfounded health risks of being within five hundred feet of an ejaculation.

Although Mayor Giuliani's crusade undoubtedly made it difficult for professional masturbators to continue legally operating within the city's entertainment districts, the rise of the internet in the mid- to late 1990s arguably had a bigger impact on the decline of the in-person peep show.

The Digital-Era Peep Show

By the turn of the twenty-first century, peep show establishments were beginning to be viewed as relics of a bygone era. "These still exist?" utter amused tourists entering sexually oriented businesses and seeing booths reserved for in-person private shows. This sentiment, coupled with continued stereotypes and misinformation about the health risks of "sticky floors," has made the demand for in-person masturbation shows minimal. In its place came the rise of camming, the "digital-era peep show."

Camming can include stripteases, masturbation, and partnered sex acts on an online platform where customers can view performances, chat with performers, and pay for sexually explicit shows. As a form of sex work, and in particular online sex work, camming is often shrugged off as not "real work." There is a false perception that camming is easy money and that anyone can earn a living from masturbating in front of a webcam. This myth strips away the skills needed to market oneself to an identified target audience to make enough money to pay for DoorDash deliveries, let alone to earn enough to make a career out of it.

Performer Demi Sutra, for example, has over 700,000 followers across social media platforms like Twitter, Instagram, and TikTok. She's a top earner on OnlyFans with over a quarter of a million likes on her thousands of masturbation pictures, videos, and live-stream camming sessions. Sutra markets herself nearly constantly on these platforms to stay engaged with her fans, occasionally even dressing up as Cat Woman or Princess Leia to cater to the nerds and geeks in her audience. This amount of work is anything but "easy money" that anyone can do.

Camming is a form of independent contracting or freelance labor that requires significant effort, but also affords the worker greater flexibility than a traditional nine-to-five office job. But for the skeptics who are not convinced that online sex work is real work, "real work" apparently requires a boss, a forced schedule, permission slips to be sick, and the excruciating pain of feigning interest during staff meetings.

If you are getting paid for it, including getting paid to masturbate, it's work.

Apart from the ridiculous labor definition gatekeeping, online sex workers are also faced with the stigma of being in a profession that is viewed as immoral, degrading, perverse, and any other pejorative Ben Shapiro uses to describe rap music.

There is a belief that online sex workers are being exploited or are exploiting themselves, to which many cam workers have countered with their own narratives that are defined by personal empowerment. But it is a false dichotomy to view sex work as being either inherently exploitative or inherently empowering. Sociology professor Dr. Ronald Weitzer said that sex work is composed of a "constellation of occupational arrangements, power relations, and worker experiences," meaning that sex work, like all work, is complex and cannot be thought of in simple terms as being either 100 percent exploitative or 100 percent empowering for everyone all the time. Terms like *degrading* and *empowerment* are subjective feelings for every worker and are not solely tied to one job. Nevertheless, there is a holier-than-thou double standard placed upon sex workers and sex work. It is easy to cast stones at a criminalized and stigmatized job while ignoring your own exploitation at the hands of your bosses. For those who think all sex work is degrading, I'm assuming the Monday morning commute to a cubicle is full of happiness and empowerment.

Pointing out this double standard, someone will inevitably think, *Well, I'd much prefer working in an office than [insert sex work stereotype or overly graphic description of violence].*

Okay.

Thanks for sharing.

You may feel degraded if you were a sex worker. But not everyone does. You may feel empowered working as an accountant. But not everyone does. We don't expect every worker to be happy with their job and to feel empowered by it, but we place that unrealistic expectation on sex workers in order to "legitimize" their work.

No one should have to work a job they do not want to do. No one should have to work if they do not want to. That should be the goal, but that is not the current reality. What is not helpful are moral judgments about work you personally disapprove of. What is helpful is working collectively to improve labor conditions for the workers in your industry, and to support other workers in their own organizing efforts to do the same.

Getting Paid to Have Orgasms

Dr. Angela Jones, a sociology professor at Farmingdale State College in New York and author of the 2020 book *Camming: Money, Power, and Pleasure in the Sex Work Industry*, is the leading academic expert in the area of camming. Beginning in 2013, Dr. Jones conducted a five-year, mixed-method sociological study focused on camming and the camming industry, reporting on the nuanced and diverse experiences of professional masturbators in online spaces.

Based on Dr. Jones's surveys and interviews, many cam workers report sexual pleasure as being a benefit of their job. One worker learned how to masturbate to orgasm for the first time because her job allowed her to become more comfortable with her body. Another worker said that masturbating for a living made it easier for her to reach orgasm with a partner during sex. In terms of feeling degraded by the work, one cam worker stated, "If you're talking about camming . . . I'm empowered by it . . . I get paid to have orgasms. That's fucking legit."

However, the downsides and risks of camming include *capping* (short for capturing), which is a tactic used by cam show viewers to record live shows, either for personal use, to upload onto third-party porn sites, or for blackmail. Despite this theft, cam workers have often resigned to this unethical behavior, thinking that it is "pretty much inevitable."

Another danger is doxing through oversharing personal information, identifiable scenery in the background of their cam room, or getting their computer hacked, all of which can lead to in-person stalking, harassment, and threats of violence. But even if in-person harassment is avoided through protecting personal information, cam workers who participated in Dr. Jones's research reported regular instances of online harassment from internet trolls. Cam workers often navigate this risk and harassment by ignoring the trolls and reducing them to having "internet tough guy syndrome." For one cam worker who was annoyed, but ultimately not threatened by trolls, she believes "It's posturing; they talk big game but most of them can't even muster the give-a-shit to go to the grocery store. They're self-entitled shut-ins."

A part of this polymorphous paradigm within camming is discrimination based on age, race, and body size. Whereas porn companies and in-person peep show businesses may have implicit (and sometimes explicit) discriminatory hiring practices, camming is open to anyone with a webcam, thus eliminating the approval of a masturbation gatekeeper only interested in young, white, and thin cam workers. And although prejudice and discrimination still exist in the camming world, such as Black workers earning less than their white peers, it is nevertheless still viewed as more diverse than other spaces within the sex industry.

Racism, ageism, and fatphobia in camming create a dilemma for marginalized workers who must decide whether they want to fight against stereotypes and fetishization within the industry or to exploit them for profit. According to Dr. Jones's research, some workers quit camming because of this, whereas others tolerate it for the money or even fully embrace it.

With body size, for example, some workers reported concerns about their weight getting fetishized and their entire identity getting reduced to the category "BBW" (big beautiful women).[50] But other workers found this categorization empowering, as one woman stated, "Camming does more to speak to my inner Goddess than to fuel my insecurity. Men love me. Men pay for me." For others, weight fetishization is not viewed as exploitative or empowering, but simply a way to get paid, with one cam worker noting, "My fat ass makes me money, my tummy banks with $9-per-minute exclusive shows."

Who could argue with that?

Commercializing Circle Jerks

Male cam workers were also part of Dr. Jones's research, often citing the same motivations, benefits, and risks of the job as women performers. Although one man reported "getting to masturbate for a paycheck is still

---

50. In 2012, fragrance company Bath & Body Works had fragrance testing strips in their stores branded with their new slogan, "I ♥ BBW," presumably unaware that they were promoting body inclusivity alongside eucalyptus spearmint essential oil.

pretty cool," the sex industry is one of the few labor industries where there is an inverted wage gap, with women outearning men. With the earning potential low, pleasure was more important than pay for one seventy-year-old male cam worker in Dr. Jones's study who reported, "I like to masturbate, and I like to be watched." For these exhibitionists who are less concerned about being able to pay rent by ejaculating in front of strangers, social media may be a better platform than cam sites.

In a kink blink, social media was sexualized with the creation of websites catering to users' interests in sharing sexually explicit photos and videos that would otherwise violate the terms of service on Facebook. Dubbed as a "worldwide masturbation community," BateWorld is one such social media site, where users can upload and browse photos of penises, anuses, and masturbating penises and anuses. While your boss may be annoyed with how much time you spend on Instagram and TikTok, accessing BateWorld on your work computer during company time will likely result in a meeting with HR.[51]

Like most social media platforms, signing up and using its basic features like sharing photos, reading blog posts, and joining discussions in the forums are free. But for those looking for a more immersive masturbatory experience, memberships can be purchased to bring masturbation into an online commercial space. With purchasing plans ranging from $12 a month to a more economical $60 a year, paying members can upload and view masturbation videos, and can go cam-to-cam with strangers to indulge in a digital circle jerk.

Unlike cam sites that are structured with a client paying a sex worker to masturbate, BateWorld's fees go to the site's administrators who maintain and permit access to an online space where you can pay

---

51. BateWorld can only be accessed from a computer. Apple and Google do not allow a BateWorld app in a vain attempt to appear as moral and ethical companies.

to "amp up your penis pleasure with your brothers in bate." It's non-hierarchical, communal cumming.

The space is further commercialized with ads and its own Bate-Shop offering a variety of masturbation accessories like lube, vibrators, and cock rings. BateWorld, like camming sites, has masturbatory appeal for its accessibility and many options of anonymity. However, for those wanting a real-life experience of communal masturbation, jack-off clubs may be the analog masturbation experience you've been craving in the digital age.

Jack-Off Clubs

While in-person peep shows may have experienced a decline in demand with the rise of camming, jack-off clubs[52] is one sector of the masturbation industry that has maintained its popularity over the past several decades.

Men masturbating around other men is a millennia-old pastime and has even been sung about in a nineteenth-century Scottish folk song ("The elders of the church, they were too old to firk, so they sat around the table and had a circle jerk"). But the quasi-commercialization of this communal experience can be traced to the 1970s during the rise of the gay rights movement and solidified in 1980 with the founding of New York Jacks, the first masturbation club.

Quickly expanding to other cities beginning with San Francisco Jacks in 1983 (and dozens after, including Denver, Atlanta, Toronto, London, and Madrid), jack-off clubs not only provided a space for masturbation fetishists and those desiring communal masturbation, but also a safe sexual outlet during the height of the AIDS epidemic in the 1980s.

---

52. For the grammar nerds, *jack-off* is an adjective, *jack off* is a verb, and *jackoff* is a derogatory noun. Used in a sentence, "I don't want to jack off next to any jackoffs at the jack-off club."

By having the standard rules of "No lips below the hips" and "Nothing goes inside anybody's anything," jack-off clubs offer parameters of sexual behavior that skirt HIV and most STI transmission.

Jack-off clubs are distinct from bathhouses, where the latter offers an environment for a variety of sexual behaviors, and the former is restricted to mutual masturbation. During the AIDS epidemic, New York City put pressure on the city's bathhouses, deeming them a public health risk, despite little evidence supporting the contention that sexual behaviors within the bathhouses were contributing to widespread community transmission of HIV. But much like the peep shows in Times Square, any establishment of public ejaculation is stereotyped as a vector of disease.

Jack-off clubs, on the other hand, have largely operated underground, without a consistent brick-and-mortar presence that would subject it to the moralizing crusades of elected officials and their misguided zoning ordinances.

Paul Rosenberg, a former professional singer and corporate worker at Starbucks who founded Rain City Jacks in Seattle in 2005, told me in an email exchange, "Since few places in the United States specifically accommodate sex parties, the majority of Jacks simply operate in the shadows." Club events are typically held in rented spaces that usually serve other erotic purposes, like BDSM clubs, back rooms of gay bars, erotic art galleries, hotel rooms, and private homes. One club in Arkansas held events in a motel next to a Hobby Lobby and a Walmart, which made the communal jacking off the healthiest and most ethical thing happening in that strip mall.

If the event site is targeted by a busybody, future events are just moved to another location the next month. It is a moving target for the anti-masturbation crusaders, with the bators always one step ahead in their quest to freely masturbate in the company of like-minded bros.

Like BateWorld, the monetization of masturbation exists to cover the costs of providing a space for mutual masturbators. At Rain City Jacks, for example, access to this private space requires membership fees ranging from $20 trials to $225 all-you-can-jack annual dues. According to Rosenberg, most jack-off clubs operate as nonprofits. Membership fees just make sure the events are functional and cover such services as individual lube, antibacterial moist wipes, venue rental fees, and liability insurance in case someone trips over an erection.

Jacking Rules

Beyond the basic rules of no blow jobs and butt stuff, jack-off clubs have a long list of rules for attendees to abide by in order to ensure a pleasurable masturbation experience for all.

"Excessive chatter" is discouraged to avoid killing the masturbatory vibe with dull conversation about Raisin Bran and colonoscopies. No alcohol or drugs are permitted, and no one should have a communicable disease like an active herpes outbreak, flu, or staph infection. Also, under no circumstances should a member identify another member outside of the club. Anonymity and discretion are stressed at jack-off clubs, operating with similar rules as Fight Club.

There is also a list of ejaculation etiquette that includes verbally announcing when you're about to climax and not just implying it by heavily breathing. Semen is allowed on yourself, canvas-covered furniture, and the floor.[53] Semen is never allowed on someone else's face or anus, but backs, thighs, and elbows are fine. Ingesting semen from any surface or directly from the source is also prohibited, but some clubs provide non-semen snacks to satisfy any hunger cravings.

---

53. Shoes are required at club events.

Explicit consent and mutual respect govern the space at jack-off clubs. Although masturbation is the central focus, club attendees can touch each other under certain conditions. Any kissing, nipple rubbing, or touching another member's member is prohibited unless given verbal consent. However, an exception to verbal consent is wearing a green wristband, which indicates anyone can touch your penis without asking permission first. Wearing a red wristband indicates you do not want your penis touched. Wearing two red wristbands is homophobic.

Considering the fee and the plethora of rules, many may question what even is the appeal of masturbating at a jack-off club. In an article for *GQ* discussing the phenomenon of "buddy bating," writer Ej Dickson noted the intimacy and self-empowerment that accompanies guys masturbating in front of other guys, as one bator noted, "And while some might argue that a group of dudes masturbating on drop cloth–covered furniture doesn't exactly constitute an emotional connection, taking an act that is as solitary and intimate and so traditionally laden with shame as masturbation and making it communal can be transformative."

Writer John Sherman published a story about a first-time experience of attending a jack-off club in 2018 for *BuzzFeed News*. He reported how the guys in attendance at an event hosted by New York Jacks viewed masturbation as ". . . an experience to be sought for its own sake" instead of viewing it as a subpar replacement for partnered sex. One of the organizers for the event said, "Masturbating with other guys takes away much of our culture's shame and embarrassment about this universal practice." For others, though, it's less about self-empowerment and more about having something to do on a day off like "a free-time activity featuring penises."

Similarly, when *The Stranger* staff writer Christopher Frizzelle explored the topic in 2019 at Rain City Jacks, one member told him it is an enjoyable, weekly routine. "It's wholesome, clean fun," he said. "It's like going to church for me on Sunday."

No Homo

When one thinks of a guy paying a monthly membership fee for the privilege of masturbating with a bunch of other guys, heterosexuality isn't a word that usually comes to mind. However, the desire to masturbate in a room full of penises can transcend any particular sexual orientation.

According to Rosenberg, approximately 10 percent of members of Rain City Jacks are straight men. This aligns with data from BateWorld, where 10 percent of the site's seventy thousand users are heterosexual. On the surface, it would be easy to interpret this statistic as meaning 10 percent of jack-off club and BateWorld members are closeted gay men, or at least closeted bisexual men.

But a heterosexual orientation and being turned on by masturbating in the company of other men are not incompatible if you consider all of the reasons that such behavior might be arousing. For some, it is fetishistic, where the object of sexual arousal is the penis, regardless of who it is attached to. For others, it is exhibitionistic, where the sexual arousal stems from masturbating in front of someone else, regardless of the gender of the observer. And for some others, it can simply be a nostalgic male bonding experience. Considering that this behavior is common among adolescent boys where upwards of 20 percent of teens have reported masturbating with their guy friends,[54] the straight jack-off club member may be longing for a shared experience with his male friends that is generally frowned upon on a golf course.

Additionally, it may be arousing for men to watch other men masturbate because they know what it feels like to rub their own penis. It's less about voyeurism and more about empathy. Seeing someone else

---

54. A not-too-uncommon game among adolescents in the UK is called *soggy biscuit*, where teen boys race to ejaculate onto a biscuit and the last one to finish has to eat it. A reminder to parents to always knock before entering your son's bedroom.

masturbate can conjure up feelings of shared pleasure from understanding the sensations when seeing semen hit the floor.

But most simply, shared masturbation may just be the result of being a masturbation enthusiast. If you have a desire to masturbate, and are surrounded by people just as excited as you and are encouraging you, sexual orientation doesn't really matter. As Dickson quoted a straight bator in her *GQ* article, ". . . most men, regardless of sexual orientation, really love their penises. And they love to masturbate."

It can be as simple as that.

CHAPTER 9

'Til Death Do Us Part

Successful Aging, Assisted Living, and Romantic Necrophilia

D r. Emery C. Abbey, a urological surgeon from Buffalo, New York, warned the public of the dangers of self-pleasure in his pamphlet, *The Sexual System and Its Derangements*. In the pamphlet, published in 1875, he discussed how masturbation was incompatible with successful aging and the most destructive sin that will inevitably lead to "premature decay . . . until death is reached." He believed that if someone was unable to curb their sexual appetite for self-defilement, it would hasten the masturbator "into a premature grave, loaded with violent forms of disease, with debasement of the human soul and the mind filled with obscenity and beastliness."

From a supposed area of medical expertise, Dr. Abbey believed a "great majority of the ills of humanity arise directly from the injury done by self-abuse." Dr. Abbey thought having an orgasm and ejaculating were so shocking to the body's nervous system that preventing orgasm was critical in promoting health. He warned readers to be vigilant and wary of the various ways one can inadvertently have an orgasm, such as from riding horseback,[55] being in the presence of a woman, listening to lewd stories, and by "straining at stool."

---

55. This is in contrast to what Dr. Benjamin Rush (from chapter 4) suggested, arguing that long journeys on horseback *decrease* masturbatory desire. Rest assured, equestrians, neither assertion is true.

By citing the Bible as an example of how men could live over a hundred years by living purely, Dr. Abbey promised he could restore a prematurely aging masturbator to live a life of vitality. He devoted over five hundred words to explaining the greatness of his medicinal cure for onanism and how it will reduce sexual desire so retained semen can be reabsorbed to "vivify [a person] with new life and energy."

Claiming to have sold 500,000 copies at ten cents apiece, Dr. Abbey's pamphlet did not offer specifics of what the medicine is or what it actually does. He only mentioned that it derives from "a common plant" and that it will not disrupt the masturbator's life with nausea. He makes bold claims that his cure hasn't disappointed him in five years and that it is a remedy "with a success never before achieved." It promises to "allay unnatural sexual desire so that masturbation is repulsive" and the sufferer should be cured within one month's time. But despite the lack of pharmacological details, Dr. Abbey would mail you this plant-based cure to reverse the prematurely aging effects of masturbation for the low cost of $10. It was the nineteenth-century purity version of today's anti-aging creams.

The Aging Orgasm

Dr. Abbey's beliefs are rejected by the medical community today as nothing more than quackery, but his attitudes about the incompatibility of masturbation and successful aging are still widespread in our culture. Like children, older adults are stripped of their unique sexuality and are perceived as people devoid of sexual thoughts, feelings, and behaviors. This ageist belief holds that older adults spend their retirement eating Müeslix and playing backgammon, not sitting on a suction-cupped dildo scrolling thirst traps.

Which is why the hosts of Fox News's morning show, *Fox & Friends*, were shocked to learn the secret of aging according to ninety-one-year-old actor Ernest Borgnine during a 2008 interview. Borgnine, whose career spanned six decades, is most memorable from roles in *From Here to Eternity*, *Marty* (earning him an Oscar), and *McHale's Navy*. Beginning in his eighties, he was the voice of the Mermaid Man on *SpongeBob SquarePants*. On- and off-screen, he had the persona of a lovable and loving grandpa. And when asked what the secret of aging is, the Academy Award–winning nonagenarian leaned toward host Steve Doocy and whispered, "I masturbate a lot."

The Fox morning team burst into an uncomfortable laughter, covered their embarrassed faces, and quickly cut to commercial. Although it doesn't take much to get a strong emotional reaction from Fox News hosts when discussing anything sexual, the response is not atypical as it relates to older adult masturbation.

Teaching college students about older adult sexuality often elicits similar reactions of discomfort and disgust. The intrusive thought of their grandparents using vibrators and sex dolls is often too much to tolerate in class on a Thursday afternoon.

To counter this knee-jerk reaction of disapproval, I try to have my students broaden their perspective of aging sexuality, and even personalize it. I will ask at what age do they no longer want to masturbate. Taken aback by the question and being confronted with imagining their own trajectory into older adulthood, the young adults recognize that it wouldn't be ideal to have to trade in masturbation for a senior discount at Chick-fil-A.

The reality is that older adults, typically defined as those sixty-five years old and older, masturbate. Although prevalence rates may range from 10 to 90 percent, data suggests that approximately 60 percent of older men and 30 to 45 percent of older women report masturbating in the past year. As with younger adults, masturbation is less preferred than partnered sex, and masturbation frequency among older adults is inversely related to the religious conservatism of a country or culture. Dr. Bente Træen, a psychology professor from the University of Oslo, examined cross-cultural differences in masturbation between northern and southern European countries. Unsurprisingly, in the more religiously conservative Portugal, only 42 percent of older adult men and 27 percent of older adult women reported masturbating in the past month. This compares to 65 percent of older adult men and 40 percent of older adult women in the more secular Norway.[56]

In a 2007 study published in the *New England Journal of Medicine*, the researchers noted a decrease in masturbation frequency with age, with those in the oldest-old cohort (over eighty-five years old) reporting the lowest frequency. However, age in and of itself may not be the best predictor of declining desire to masturbate. Jokes are aplenty about sagging breasts and pendulous scrotums among the elderly, but age-related gravity does not diminish the capacity for pleasure.

Declining health, however, particularly experiencing diseases and disabilities that directly impact sexual functioning, can significantly lower masturbation occurrence. Considering that sexual functioning requires healthy neurological, hormonal, muscular, and vascular systems, aging increases the likelihood that one of those bodily systems will be impacted by disease or injury, thus making masturbation more challenging or less satisfying.

While there are various medications that can directly or indirectly assist with sexual functioning, the aging masturbator will also need to make changes to their expectations and behaviors. What worked for someone's masturbation routine in their twenties won't necessarily work for them in their seventies. Older adults may need to change positions,

---

56. Norway is consistently rated as having the highest quality of life and being the "happiest place on Earth." The country's tourism officials are missing an opportunity to advertise how masturbation may be a cause or consequence of that.

use more lube, increase the speed or pressure on their vibrator, have fewer distractions, and, most importantly, have more patience if they want to masturbate to orgasm.

Long gone may be the days of sneaking off to the bathroom for a quick ninety-second orgasm in between conference calls. Older adult masturbation may require more intention and more planning, but that does not mean it comes at the price of satisfaction. In fact, masturbation is not only reported to be satisfying in and of itself, but it is related to higher levels of life satisfaction, especially for single older adults without a sexual partner. Physical changes are a part of aging, and so may be changes in our environments that would require masturbatory adaptations as well.

Some Privacy, Please

Older adult masturbation, as a taboo behavior, lives in the shadows. That is, of course, until a beam of light is cast into the shadow from an aide opening an elderly person's door at a nursing home.

When older adults rely on additional living assistance and move into long-term care facilities, it comes at the expense of sexual privacy. No longer afforded the freedom to masturbate whenever and wherever in the comfort of their own home, older adults in care facilities now have to navigate communal living spaces where masturbating openly would disrupt the rules of Taco Tuesday in the dining hall.

This navigation requires strategies to ensure privacy in communal living settings and to reduce the likelihood of getting caught with your pants down—both are similar to the strategies that were employed decades earlier during childhood and adolescence. And as during youth, the consequences of getting caught masturbating will vary depending on who is doing the intruding. Long-term care facilities typically do not have policies that explicitly prohibit or promote masturbation, leaving the acceptability of the behavior dependent on the sexual attitudes of the staff. Dr. Feliciano Villar, a psychology professor and aging specialist at the University of Barcelona, researched these attitudes in a series of studies from 2016 to 2018.

Data from the studies revealed that masturbation was the most commonly observed sexual behavior in long-term care facilities, and it was also the behavior that made the staff the most uncomfortable. Some staff members reported worrying that other people would be offended and disgusted by accidentally walking in on an older adult masturbating. For others, surprise was the emotion most reported, with one staff member commenting, "I'd be taken aback . . . because it seems that at that age you can't do it any more, I mean, it's hard to imagine that you'd still feel like that."

But not all staff held discriminatory or ignorant attitudes about older adults masturbating. Most felt that the behavior is a private matter that should be respected, recognizing that the long-term care facility is their new home. One staff member reported feeling bad for intruding on the privacy of a masturbating older adult, stating, "Poor guy, I've interrupted him with the job half done."

And for the most sexually progressive staff members from Dr. Villar's research, they viewed it as their professional responsibility not only to respect the masturbating older adult's privacy, but to fetch them lube if the resident desired.

However, a complicating matter for staff in long-term care facilities is when an older adult resident has a neurocognitive disorder, like Alzheimer's disease. Within the medical and psychological fields, the intersection of sexuality and dementia typically focuses on partnered sex and the capacity to consent, but support staff are more likely confronted with an older adult with dementia who is masturbating in inappropriate places like dining halls and shared living spaces.

Support staff and administration are in the position to balance sexual freedom of the individual and safety of the other residents who may not desire to have an episode of *The Price Is Right* interrupted by Dolores masturbating two rocking chairs over. For chronic rule violators, long-term care administrators will need to inform the resident's adult children that their parent may get evicted for being a public masturbator.

Unfortunately, much like the sadistic cruelty of Dr. Kellogg's recommendations for curbing masturbation in children, there have been numerous punitive strategies employed to reduce masturbation in older adults, such as scolding, binding them in hard-to-remove clothing, and using prescription hormones. But just as with children, these techniques and methods are inhumane, cruel, and unnecessary. The goal is not to eliminate masturbation in older adults, but to encourage them to recognize that it needs to be done in appropriate places. There are plenty of ethical strategies that can be utilized by support staff that can redirect the older adult to masturbate in private and not on the billiards table in the rec room.

A Dying Wish

When an older adult receives a terminal prognosis, palliative care is often initiated to optimize comfort during their remaining weeks or months of life. From pain management to praying with a chaplain to watching reruns of a favorite sitcom, older adults are able to dictate an environment that best suits their dying needs. However, sexual needs have historically been an overlooked area of comfort within palliative care.

Dr. Kate Morrissey Stahl, a clinical associate professor of social work at the University of Georgia, recognized this dearth of attention to the sexual expression needs of older adults in palliative care. In 2017, she and her colleagues published guidelines in the journal *OMEGA* to help those in the social work field to better serve and advocate for the sexual needs of palliative care patients. Focusing on multiple levels of intervention, including the individual, familial, institutional, and cultural, Dr. Morrissey Stahl recognized the need for older adults to create a "loving will" that outlines their desires for sexual expression at the end of their life.

Focusing on masturbation, this may include getting prescribed medications that can assist in sexual functioning. It may include having access to lubricants, sex toys, and pornography. It may involve family members or staff at long-term care facilities providing these resources and making sure vibrators and laptops are fully charged when needed. Additional assistance may be necessary to help the older adult get into a comfortable position, physically handing them their vibrator, and pushing play on their favorite squirting video on PornHub.

Experts such as Dr. Eli Coleman, the former director of the Institute for Sexual and Gender Health at the University of Minnesota Medical School, considers masturbation to be a pillar of overall sexual health and well-being. Therefore, incorporating masturbation into end-of-life care is acknowledging that sexual quality of life is tied to overall quality of life. However, there is research to support that sexual satisfaction with a partner is a better predictor of overall life satisfaction than simply masturbation. But the research also shows that non-partnered masturbation is better tied to well-being than abstinence, suggesting that any orgasm is better than no orgasm.

But if masturbating close to death becomes impractical or no longer a priority, having strangers masturbate on your behalf can be life's final rite of passage. As was the case when ninety-year-old masturbation pioneer Betty Dodson entered into a long-term care facility in 2020 for palliative management of liver failure. With only months to live, Dodson's popular BodySex workshops were taken over by her longtime collaborator, Carlin Ross, who moved the sessions online via Zoom during the COVID-19 pandemic. But unlike Zoom meetings at the *New Yorker*, masturbation was encouraged for all meeting attendees.

Daily Beast writer Stephanie Theobald attended one of these online BodySex workshops in August of that year. Theobald reported that Ross wanted to create an experience to honor her friend and told the women in the Zoom workshop that they were going to collectively offer their "orgasm energy today to Betty's transition."

Dodson, not shying away from the reality she was facing, believed that "we need to embrace death like it's our final orgasm." Upon learning about the masturbatory Zoom classes in her honor, Dodson said, "Good. That's what I want." A dying wish to be celebrated with masturbation after a lifetime of teaching the celebration of masturbating.

No longer limited to a small circle of women in a Manhattan apartment, crowded around a shared outlet for Magic Wand vibrators, Theobald reported that dozens of eager women from all over the world were logging into the Zoom session, ready to pay their respects to a woman who has liberated their masturbation.

The collective thumbnail faces of grimaces and groans provided the most appropriate salute to one of the field's mavericks. On whether a group of masturbating women is actually providing any sort of comfort to a dying woman, Theobald argued that if Christians believe prayers can offer help to those close to death, why can't orgasms?

Dodson later died on Halloween of that year. Eulogizing her friend, legendary artist and former porn performer Annie Sprinkle said of Dodson, "She was always the life, and clitoris, of the party."

Memento Mori

From research about older adults masturbating, the one factor that increases the frequency of masturbation is the death of a spouse or partner. This increase is primarily due to now relying on masturbation as

DIY

the sole sexual outlet, but the increase is also due to coping with grief. Masturbation and orgasm can provide momentary pleasure and relief from the sadness during periods of mourning. However, feelings of guilt about masturbating after the death of a loved one are common. What is an appropriate mourning period of abstinence? What is the etiquette of having an orgasm a month after the funeral? A week after the funeral? During the funeral?

This sense of guilt is often rooted in the same irrational belief about the function of masturbation within a relationship. There are concerns that the solitary act is cheating or disrespectful toward your partner. A belief that your sexuality should only be directed toward the person you love, and not yourself. If masturbation was viewed as uniquely ours, then only grief, not guilt, would be an inhibiting factor to masturbating after a loss.

There is no right or wrong time to masturbate after the death of a loved one. Since masturbation serves so many different functions, a person may have zero interest in masturbating for many weeks or months. For others, masturbation could offer comfort and at least a fleeting moment of pleasure. It may afford an opportunity for escapism by fantasizing about the fling you had during the summer of 1985 when your boyfriend went down on you in a theater during a screening of *The Breakfast Club*.

For others, they may want to masturbate in honor of a dead spouse, reminiscing on the fun and pleasurable times they shared. They may scroll through old sexts and nudes, sniff their clothing, and incorporate other mementos into their masturbation. Much like the function of a shrine, it is in an attempt to honor and reconnect with their partner.[57]

---

57. Check your local public indecency laws about masturbating in a cemetery if your shrine is at their burial site.

And for those who want an even more immersive experience, Jade Stanley of Bromsgrove, England, made salacious headlines in the British tabloids in 2018 after it was learned that her business was selling personally crafted sex dolls made to look like your deceased spouse. In an interview with the *Sun*, Stanley stated that she wanted "to help people that are seeking comfort" during their grieving process. "It can be very beneficial for them," she said, "and helps them keep a piece of their loved one; it provides them with comfort and people don't always buy the dolls for a sordid reason."

Although it is perfectly healthy to buy a dead lover replica even for "sordid" reasons, the public was not impressed. Armchair grief counselors on Twitter opined that masturbating with a sex doll that resembles your dead loved one would prolong the stages of grief. Aside from the fact the stages of grief are not empirically sound, and grief is not a universal or linear process, why would this masturbatory act prolong grief? How is it different than "hanging on" to any number of behaviors that a grieving widow engages in to honor the memory of their former partner?

Admittedly, masturbating with a sex doll that resembles a dead lover may sound strange or even deeply unsettling and disturbing to many. It is certainly not a common mourning practice found in any culture. However, a good number of mourning rituals throughout the world are often considered unsettling and disturbing to outside observers. In Japan, for example, there is a phone booth in Otsuchi with a disconnected black rotary phone where mourners can have "conversations" with their deceased loved ones. In Brazil, up until the 1960s, the Wari people used to eat their loved ones in order to process their grief and to diminish the intensity of the memories of the dead. In Indonesia, the Torajan people keep the mummified corpses of their loved ones in their homes for years after death. Even after the bodies are eventually placed in tombs, surviving family members still clean and care for the deceased, often changing their clothing and providing them with gifts.

Just because something is unsettling, offensive, or disturbing to you doesn't mean it is unhealthy for others to practice.

But if the thought of staring into plastic eyes would be more depressing than arousing, Dutch designer Mark Sturkenboom has a subtler option for romantic necrophilia.

In 2015, Sturkenboom designed a wooden memory box that opens with a brass key and includes small drawers for keepsakes like a ring, a speaker for an iPhone to play their favorite tunes, and a diffuser for perfume or cologne, all designed to give the grieving widow or widower a chance to relive sensory memories of their deceased partner. But the selling point of this box is a gold-plated urn inside a glass dildo that can hold twenty-one grams[58] of cremated ashes.

Inspired by taboo sexuality and the oft-loveless display of cremains in traditional urns, Sturkenboom wanted to "open a new window for the way we reminisce about someone and find a dialogue for these feelings people are struggling with when somebody passes."

Although it is unknown if any purchases of Sturkenboom's vibrator urn are bought for the novelty or with the earnest intent of masturbating with cremains, it nonetheless showcases the possibilities of integrating masturbation, grief, and death.

Whether the anti-masturbation hucksters want to admit it or not, masturbation is part of the human experience from birth to death. As long as you desire it, there is no reason to abstain from masturbating

---

58. Twenty-one grams was intentionally selected based on the debunked claim that the human body loses twenty-one grams of weight at the moment of death, suggesting that is the weight of the soul. Any decrease in weight at the moment of death is attributed to the loss of air or gas from the lungs or anus. Strangely, this fact has yet to turn into a claim arguing that the soul is actually farted into the afterlife.

up until the moment of your last heartbeat. And while death brings the end of your pleasure, there may be some solace in knowing that your memory will be part of others' masturbatory fantasies for years to come.

Much like Betty Dodson, we can strive to leave a legacy of orgasms.

Conclusion

Masturbation Liberation, Self-Care, and Happy Endings

The first generation of feminist sex shops focused on collective liberation through masturbation. Dell Williams, founder of Eve's Garden, which opened in 1974 in New York, viewed masturbation as a way for women to become more in touch with their autonomy and their own power. In turn, this would allow them to utilize that power politically. The stores offered physical space for community events that focused on educating customers about their bodies and how sex toys offered a path to sexual and gender liberation. Masturbation liberation was considered a first step in revolutionizing the world.

Over time, however, sexually oriented retail shops expanded and franchised. In order to stay in business, they became less about community engagement and more about profit. The sexual revolution, as it pertains to masturbation, shifted from collective liberation to individual empowerment to a hyper-commercialization of pleasure and wellness that has eager masturbators bargain shopping on Amazon to get a cheap vibrator delivered by 10 p.m. for "me time."

This shift coincided with an emerging wellness industry that has turned public health into individual consumer choices. Much like the medicine shows of yore, current wellness companies offer a host of products and services with guarantees of a better life. For the right price, you can purchase your way to smoother skin, greater longevity, and a stronger vagina.

One such company, Goop, started in 2018 by Academy Award–winning actress Gwyneth Paltrow, offers consumers workout accessories (like a $55 jump rope), "detox" diets, gold-plated vibrating rollers to sculpt your face, and an egg-shaped jade stone that is designed to be held in your vagina. The egg was originally advertised with promises to "increase vaginal muscle tone, hormonal balance, and feminine energy in general." For the price of $66,[59] you could improve your health by walking around town with a rock in your vagina.

But, Dr. Jen Gunter, an ob-gyn and author of *The Vagina Bible,* who has a long history of calling out pseudoscience as it relates to women's health, was no fan of Paltrow's vaginal eggs. In a blog post on her website in 2017, Dr. Gunter dismissed the claims, particularly ones about the eggs impacting hormones, as "the biggest load of garbage."

State prosecutors in California agreed and filed a lawsuit accusing Goop of making unscientific claims about the eggs and other products. In 2018, Goop settled the suit by agreeing to pay $145,000 in civil penalties and offering refunds to consumers who felt duped by the proclaimed curative power of a "yoni egg."

Despite the lawsuit and its settlement, Goop hasn't shied away from continuing its quest to sell sexual wellness products and promote sexual pleasure. Listed next to vibrators and herbal supplements called "Desire Gummies," the jade eggs are still for sale on Goop's website, but are now advertised to offer non-specific (i.e., California state law–approved) health benefits like "crystal healing" and encouraging buyers to "harness the power of energy work." Possibly to ensure effectiveness or longevity of the eggs, the product description recommends the eggs be stored in a place that has "good vibes."

---

59. Or "four interest-free payments of $16.50."

And to keep up with the consumer demand for wellness products and information, Goop keeps expanding, and now has produced a podcast and a Netflix docuseries called *The Goop Lab*. In addition to episodes focused on mediums communicating with the dead, energy healing, and "vampire facials"[60] to look younger, one episode in the docuseries focused on sexual pleasure and masturbation. It even featured Betty Dodson, who immediately started schooling Paltrow on the difference between a vulva and a vagina.

But much like the jade eggs, the sexual health claims made in the docuseries weren't always scientific. For example, porn was blamed for a perceived increase in women seeking plastic surgery to decrease the size of their labia, despite no evidence demonstrating that relationship. Further, the episode argues that orgasms are good for your health and can curb your appetite and increase your sense of smell, apparently giving you the powers of a bloodhound on Ozempic.

To Paltrow's credit, she is trying to help people experience more pleasure from their bodies. That part is admirable. And she's certainly not alone in this mission, nor is she alone in making exaggerated claims about the health benefits of masturbation and orgasm.

It is not uncommon for sex educators and therapists today to promote the supposed benefits of masturbation as if it were a panacea for all of life's ills. Sexual wellness influencers on TikTok and Instagram (many of whom are licensed mental health providers) regularly upload posts with bold claims about the health effects of masturbation, including how it boosts immunity, clears skin, fosters better sleep, improves body image, alleviates pain, increases self-esteem, decreases anxiety, and brings about world peace.

---

60. "Vampire facials" involve injecting plasma-rich-platelets into your face. It does not involve, at least not according to Goop, being ejaculated on by Edward from *Twilight*.

These sex educators are attempting to undo the damage caused by centuries of misinformation about masturbation that has resulted in feeling shame and guilt about self-pleasure. Ironically, however, the educators are making these claims in the same fashion as anti-masturbation crusaders by relying on misinterpretations of research and grandiose beliefs.

Many of these claims have no basis in reality, like bringing about world peace and treating acne, whereas others are based on self-reports and anecdotes. In a 2023 study published in *Archives of Sexual Behavior*, about a quarter of women and a fifth of men reported using masturbation to help them fall asleep. Given the biochemical processes involved during orgasm, there is a physical mechanism of masturbation that would explain this motivation and effect. However, 75 to 80 percent of the participants in the study did not report masturbation was used to aid in better sleep.

As with all self-reports and anecdotes, results may vary.

As masturbation liberators, we should not repeat the scientific illiteracy and hucksterism of *Onania*. We don't have to condemn masturbation as the plague of civilization, nor praise it as civilization's savior. I will not be touring the country like a twenty-first-century medicine man making exuberant and hyperbolic claims about masturbation's benefits. You will never see me in Times Square next to a depressed Elmo screaming into a megaphone, "Step right up, folks! Do you have aches and pains? Can't sleep? Always tired and cold? Constipated? Have heart disease or kidney stones? If yes, then try masturbation! The modern miracle at your fingertips!"

Work Hard, Play Hard?

Even if we rein in the exaggerated health benefits of masturbation, we must also be careful not to oversell the function of masturbation as self-care. For example, Irena Gonzalez, a columnist for *Oprah Daily*, wrote about her discovery of masturbation self-care after recognizing her insecurity about her husband's masturbatory habits. His motivation for masturbation, he told her, was less about a replacement for sex, but more about needing a quick stress relief.[61]

This piqued Gonzalez's interest because she, too, was burnt out, anxious, and unable to sleep, largely due to her stressful job. Like her husband, she learned that masturbation was an effective tool for calming down and relaxing. She was able to liberate masturbation from the irrational taboo against it within marriages and was able to engage in a pleasurable behavior that allowed her to cope with the stressors of her life.

And that's a good thing.

Much like binge-watching shows on Netflix, playing golf, and adding items to an Amazon wish list, masturbation can be an effective tool in an arsenal of stress-relieving tactics. And if it is socially acceptable to tee it up with the boys on a Saturday afternoon to cope with a sixty-hour workweek, then it should be equally acceptable to lube up your vibrator on a Friday night to do the same.

However, critics of the wellness industry argue that an emphasis on self-care ignores the origins of those stressors and puts the responsibility on the individual, not the systems, to change. By placing the burden of well-being and health on the person, we ignore the structural issues causing ill health outside of their immediate control like labor exploitation, racism, homophobia, and sexism.

The self-care message is essentially keep grinding and be productive for your boss, and HR will give you a couple of wellness tips to do on your thirty-minute lunch break.

Breathe in, breathe out.

Count to ten.

Avoid the temptation to hang yourself with your employee badge lanyard.

---

61. A clever excuse if you get caught masturbating by a disapproving partner.

Get back to work.

Self-care serves as a distraction and enough of a soothing balm to take the fuel out of any protesting for better wages and other improved working conditions. While masturbation may have temporary calming effects to deal with stress, much like any other coping strategy, it does not combat the source of the stress. The simple act of masturbation is not revolutionary.

But despite the critiques of self-care and personal wellness, self-care and collective action can coexist and be a part of the same activist and individual empowerment drive. In order to fight for liberation, one still needs to attend to their own individual needs. It's the importance of recognizing self-care not as a "treat yourself" luxury, but as a necessary behavior to continue fighting for true masturbation liberation.

Do It Yourself

Whether or not masturbation is considered a revolutionary act or just self-care, it can, nonetheless, be liberating from the bounds of traditional definitions of sex and sexual pleasure. In her book *Liberating Masturbation*, Dodson argued that masturbation allows you to become independent about sex.

If you don't have a sexual partner, you can masturbate.

If your current sexual partner is not available or not in the mood, you can masturbate.

If you feel entitled to an orgasm because of "blue balls,"[62] you can masturbate.

---

62. Blue balls, the slang term for discomfort felt in the testicles, results from prolonged blood congestion and scrotal constriction during sexual arousal. At most, it is a mild pressure put on the testes that goes away when arousal decreases. It does not cause severe pain, it is not harmful, and it is not deadly, despite what he tells you.

Masturbation liberates us to experience sexual pleasure solely on our terms and allows us to redefine sex. Either solo or partnered, it is still sex. Partnered sex is unique in its ability to have a shared experience with someone else, to feel desired, and to become vulnerable. Partnered sex, however, is not unique in its ability to provide sexual arousal, orgasm, and satisfaction.

Masturbation can do that, too. It is DIY sex.

Freeing ourselves by viewing masturbation as sex and not just something you do as a last resort when you don't have a partner allows us to experience sexual pleasure and satisfaction any time we feel like it and allows us to appreciate partnered sex for the unique non-sexual pleasure it offers.

Ultimately, however, this discourse can be viewed as just mental masturbation. It is splitting pubic hairs over the definition of sex and what constitutes liberation. The material reality, and the sole purpose of this book, is to clearly articulate the simple message that masturbation is not a bringer of disease, destruction, and death.

Masturbation is simply a moment of pleasure.

In the aforementioned 2023 study in *Archives of Sexual Behavior*, the most commonly cited reason to masturbate was "I find it pleasurable." It seems obvious when it is written in a research article, but that simple motivation to masturbate, to feel pleasure, is often overlooked or minimized. For the anti-masturbation crusaders, masturbation is viewed as being a cause or consequence of disease. For the "sex positive" grifters, masturbation is believed to be a cure. The reality, however, it is neither. It's just a brief opportunity in our stressful lives to feel good.

However, if you have no desire to masturbate, then don't. Liberating masturbation does not mean you have to masturbate with alien-shaped dildos while watching reruns of *The X-Files*. Liberating masturbation means living according to your own masturbatory desires and not interfering with others' desires (which may include masturbating with alien-shaped dildos while watching reruns of *The X-Files*).

But if you do desire to masturbate, then you should be free to do so. Free from guilt and shame. Free from health misinformation. Free from the moralistic opposition of religions, governments, quacks, hucksters, and social media busybodies.

You should be free to masturbate on your own time when you desire it. The liberty to masturbate in bed. To masturbate in the shower. To masturbate while eating corn flakes and fantasizing about flogging Dr. Kellogg.

It's your body.

It's your pleasure.

Enjoy yourself.

References

Introduction
Selling the Disease of Masturbation

Author Unknown. *Onania: Or, the Heinous Sin of Self-Pollution*. London: Pierre Varenne, 1716.

Bering, J. "One Reason Why Humans Are Special and Unique: We Masturbate. A Lot." *Scientific American*, June 22, 2010. https://blogs .scientificamerican.com/bering-in-mind/one-reason-why-humans-are -special-and-unique-we-masturbate-a-lot/.

Kellogg, J. H. *Plain Facts for Old and Young: Embracing the Natural History and Hygiene of Organic Life*. Burlington, IA: I.F. Senger and Co, 1877.

Laqueur, T. *Solitary Sex: A Cultural History of Masturbation*. Princeton, NJ: Zone Books, 2003.

Stolberg, M. "Self-Pollution, Moral Reform, and the Venereal Trade: Notes on the Sources and Historical Context of *Onania* (1716)." *Journal of the History of Sexuality* 9, nos. 1–2 (2000): 37–61.

Tissot, S. A. *L'onanisme, dissertation sur les maladies produites par la masturbation* [Onanism: A dissertation on the maladies produced by masturbation]. Paris: Lausanne, 1760.

Chapter 1
Protect the Children: Child Development, Sex Education, and Masturbating Fetuses

Armstrong, K. J., and Drabman, R. S. "Treatment of a Nine-Year-Old Girl's Public Masturbatory Behavior." *Child & Family Behavior Therapy* 20 (1998): 55–62.

Associated Press. "California's New Sex Ed Guidelines Encourage Teachers to Talk to Students about Gender Identity, Masturbation." NBC News, May 8, 2019. https://www.nbcnews.com/news/education /california-s-new-sex-ed-guidelines-encourage-teachers-talk-students -n1003596.

Bering, J. "A Baker's Dozen: Old-Fashioned Anti-Erection Gadgets for Men." *Scientific American,* December 30, 2013. https://blogs .scientificamerican.com/bering-in-mind/a-bakere28099s-dozen-old -fashioned-anti-erection-gadgets-for-men-with-illustrations/.

Bodensteiner, J. B., and Sheth, R. D. "Masturbation in Infancy and Early Childhood Presenting as a Movement Disorder." *Pediatrics (Evanston)* 117, no. 5 (2006): 1861.

Borresen, K. "8 Women Share the Stories of Their First Time Masturbating." *Huffington Post,* April 9, 2019. https://www.huffpost.com/entry /women-share-stories-first-time-masturbating_l_5cab9346e4b02 e7a705bfa8a.

Broussin, B., and Brenot, P. "Does Fetal Sexuality Exist?" *Contraception, Fertilité, Sexualité* 23, no. 11 (1995): 696–698.

Cannon, C. M. "Clinton Fires Surgeon General." *Baltimore Sun,* December 10, 1994. https://www.baltimoresun.com/news/bs-xpm-1994-12-10 -1994344068-story.html.

Cook, J. W., Altman, K., Shaw, J., and Blaylock, M. "Use of Contingent Lemon Juice to Eliminate Public Masturbation by a Severely Retarded Boy." *Behaviour Research and Therapy* 16 (1979): 131–134.

Couper, R., and Huynh, H. "Female Masturbation Masquerading as Abdominal Pain." *Journal of Paediatrics and Child Health* 38, no. 2 (2002): 199–200.

Deda, G., Çaksen, H., Suskan, E., and Gümüs, D. "Masturbation Mimicking Seizure in an Infant." *Indian Journal of Pediatrics* 68, no. 8 (2001): 779–781.

Espinoza, J. "Sex-Ed Teacher Resigns after Showing First-Graders Cartoon Video about Masturbation." *Complex*, June 13, 2021. https://amp .www.complex.com/life /dalton-school-teacher-resigns-after-teaching-first-graders-about-masturbation.

Fernandez, V., and Cajal, C. "In Utero Gratification Behaviour in Male Fetus." *Prenatal Diagnosis* 36, no. 10 (2016): 985–986.

Frankel, L. "'I've Never Thought about It': Contradictions and Taboos Surrounding American Males' Experiences of First Ejaculation (Semenarche)." *Journal of Men's Studies* 11, no. 1 (2002): 37–54.

Friedrich, W. N., Fisher, J., Broughton, D., Houston, M., and Shafran, C. R. "Normative Sexual Behavior in Children: A Contemporary Sample." *Pediatrics* 101, no. 4 (1998): 1–8.

Future of Sex Education Initiative. *National Sex Education Standards: Core Content and Skills, K–12*, 2nd ed. Washington, DC: Future of Sex Education Initiative, 2020. https://siecus.org/wp-content/uploads /2020/ 03/NSES-2020-2.pdf.

Gagnon, J. H. "Attitudes and Responses of Parents to Pre-Adolescent Masturbation." *Archives of Sexual Behavior* 14, no. 5 (1985): 451–466.

Giorgi, G., and Siccardi, M. "Ultrasonographic Observation of a Female Fetus' Sexual Behavior in Utero." *American Journal of Obstetrics and Gynecology* 175 (1996): 753.

Goldfarb, E. S., and Lieberman, L. D. "Three Decades of Research: The Case for Comprehensive Sex Education." *Journal of Adolescent Health* 68, no. 1 (2020): 13–27.

Guttmacher Institute. *Sex and HIV Education.* Washington, DC: Guttmacher Institute, 2021. https://www.guttmacher.org/state-policy/explore /sex-and-hiv-education.

Ibrahim, A., and Raymond, B. "Gratification Disorder Mimicking Childhood Epilepsy in an 18-Month-Old Nigerian Girl: A Case Report and

Review of the Literature." *Indian Journal of Psychological Medicine* 35, no. 4 (2013): 417–419.

Jan, M. M., Al Banji, M. H., and Fallatah, B. A. "Long-Term Outcome of Infantile Gratification Phenomena." *Canadian Journal of Neurological Sciences* 40, no. 3 (2013): 416–419.

Kaestle, C. E., and Allen, K. R. "The Role of Masturbation in Healthy Sexual Development: Perceptions of Young Adults." *Archives of Sexual Behavior* 40, no. 5 (2011): 983–994.

Kul, M., Baykan, H., and Kandemir, H. "A Case of Excessive Masturbation Treated with Aripiprazole." *Klinik Psikofarmakoloji Bülteni [Bulletin of Clinical Psychopharmacology]* 24, no. 1 (2014): 93–96.

Makari, G. J. "Between Seduction and Libido: Sigmund Freud's Masturbation Hypotheses and the Realignment of His Etiologic Thinking, 1897–1905." *Bulletin of the History of Medicine* 72 (1998): 638–662.

Mallants, C., and Casteels, K. "Practical Approach to Childhood Masturbation: A Review." *European Journal of Pediatrics* 167, no. 10 (2008): 1111–1117.

Martin, J., Riazi, H., Firoozi, A., and Nasiri, M. "A Sex Education Program for Teachers of Preschool Children: A Quasi-Experimental Study in Iran." *BMC Public Health* 20 (2020): 692.

McGuire, R. J., and Vallence, M. "Aversion Therapy by Electric Shock." In *Conditioning Techniques in Clinical Practice and Research,* edited by J. M. Franks, 178–188. Berlin: Springer, 1964.

Meizner, I. "Sonographic Observation of in Utero Fetal 'Masturbation.'" *Journal of Ultrasound in Medicine* 6, no. 2 (1987): 111.

Mountjoy, P. T. "Some Early Attempts to Modify Penile Erection in Horse and Human: An Historical Analysis." *Psychological Record* 24 (1974): 291–308.

REFERENCES

Omran, M. S., Ghofrani, M., and Juibary, A. G. "Infantile Masturbation and Paroxysmal Disorders." *Indian Journal of Pediatrics* 75, no. 2 (2008): 183–185.

Pavlova, E., Markov, D., Atanassova, D., Stoykova, V., and Markova, I. "Ultrasonographic Observation on Prenatal Behaviour in Male Fetuses during Second Trimester Anomaly Scan." *Ultrasound in Obstetrics and Gynecology* 54, no. S1 (2019): 408.

Rödöö, P., and Hellberg, D. "Girls Who Masturbate in Early Infancy: Diagnostics, Natural Course and a Long-Term Follow-Up." *Acta Paediatrica* 102, no. 7 (2013): 762–766.

Syfret, W. "People Tell Us about Their First Time." *Vice*, July 16, 2017. https://www.vice.com/en/article/gybmqw/people-tell-us-about -their-first-time-masturbating.

Unal, F. "Predisposing Factors in Childhood Masturbation in Turkey." *European Journal of Pediatrics* 159 (2000): 338–342.

Wagner, M. K. "A Case of Public Masturbation Treated by Operant Conditioning." *Journal of Child Psychology and Psychiatry* 9 (1968): 61–65.

World Health Organization. *International Teaching Guidance on Sexuality Education.* Paris: United Nations Educational, Scientific, and Cultural Organization, 2009. https://cdn.who.int/media/docs/default-source /reproductive-health/sexual-health/international-technical-guidance-on -sexuality-education.pdf?sfvrsn=10113efc_29&download=true.

Yang, M. L., Fullwood, E., Goldstein, J., and Mink, J. W. "Masturbation in Infancy and Early Childhood Presenting as a Movement Disorder: 12 Cases and a Review of the Literature." *Pediatrics (Evanston)* 116, no. 6 (2005): 1427–1432.

Chapter 2
Palm Sunday: Priests, Rabbis, and Satanic Masturbation

Baćak, V., and Štulhofer, A. "Masturbation among Sexually Active Young Women in Croatia: Associations with Religiosity and

193

Pornography Use." *International Journal of Sexual Health* 23, no. 4 (2011): 248–257.

Boteach, S. *Kosher Sex: A Recipe for Passion and Intimacy.* New York: Harmony, 2000.

Bullough, V. L. "Alfred Kinsey and the Kinsey Report: Historical Overview and Lasting Contributions." *Journal of Sex Research* 35, no. 2 (1998): 127–131.

Danielson, S. "Satanists' Self-Concept," Master's thesis, Minnesota State University, Mankato, 2022.

Davidson, J. K., Darling, C. A., and Norton, L. "Religiosity and the Sexuality of Women: Sexual Behavior and Sexual Satisfaction Revisited." *Journal of Sex Research* 32, no. 3 (1995): 235–243.

Dyrendal, A., Lewis, J. R., and Petersen, J. Aa. *The Invention of Satanism.* Oxford, UK: Oxford University Press, 2016.

Farley, M. *Just Love: A Framework for Christian Sexual Ethics.* New York: Continuum, 2006.

Farmer, M. A., Trapnell, P. D., and Meston, C. M. "The Relation between Sexual Behavior and Religiosity Subtypes: A Test of the Secularization Hypothesis." *Archives of Sexual Behavior* 38, no. 5 (2009): 852–865.

Honey, S. *The Devil's Tome: A Book of Modern Satanic Ritual.* Detroit, MI: Serpentïnae, 2020.

Hoseini, S. S. "Masturbation: Scientific Evidence and Islam's View." *Journal of Religion and Health* 56 (2017): 2076–2081.

Hoseini, S. S., and Gharibzadeh, S. "Squeezing the Glans Penis: A Possible Maneuver for Improving the Defecation Process and Preventing Constipation." *Medical Hypotheses* 68, no. 4 (2007): 925–926.

Human Rights Watch. "Saudi Arabia: Teachers Silenced on Blasphemy Charges." Human Rights Watch, November 16, 2005. https://www.hrw.org /news/2005/11/16/saudi-arabia-teachers-silenced-blasphemy-charges.

Kinsey, A., Pomeroy, W., and Martin, C. *Sexual Behavior in the Human Male.* Philadelphia: Saunders, 1948.

Kinsey, A., Pomeroy, W., Martin, C., and Gebhard, P. *Sexual Behavior in the Human Female.* Philadelphia: Saunders, 1953.

Kirsch, A. "Emission Standards." *Tablet,* November 20, 2019. https://www.tabletmag.com/sections/belief/articles/emission-standards-daf-yomi-285.

LaVey, A. S. *The Satanic Bible.* New York: Avon, 1969.

———. *The Satanic Rituals: Companion to The Satanic Bible.* New York: Avon, 1972.

Levada, W. "Notification on the Book *Just Love: A Framework for Christian Sexual Ethics* by Sr. Margaret A. Farley, R.S.M." Delivered in Rome, March 30, 2012, at the Sacred Congregation for the Doctrine of the Faith.

Malan, M. K., and Bullough, V. "Historical Development of New Masturbation Attitudes in Mormon Culture: Silence, Secular Conformity, Counterrevolution, and Emerging Reform." *Sexuality and Culture* 9, no. 4 (2005): 80–127.

May, W. E., Lawler, R., and Boyle, J. *Catholic Sexual Ethics: A Summary, Explanation, and Defense.* Huntington, IN: Our Sunday Visitor, 2011.

Maza, C. "Masturbation Will Make You Gay, Warns Leaked Mormon Church Document." *Newsweek,* December 14, 2017. https://www.newsweek.com/masturbation-gay-leaked-mormon-church-lgtb-religion-sex-748201.

Musagara, M. "13 Reasons Why Masturbation by a Christian Is So Dangerous." *Overcoming Satan,* July 5, 2021. https://preventsatan.com/13-reasons-why-masturbation-by-a-christian-is-so-dangerous/.

Nabbout, M. "'Masturbation Is Halal' Hashtag Goes Viral in Saudi Arabia, Sparks Debate." *StepFeed,* February 21, 2018. https://stepfeed.com

/masturbation-is-halal-hashtag-goes-viral-in-saudi-arabia-sparks-debate
-3443.

"Postal Ban Urged on Kinsey's Book." *New York Times*, August 30,
1953. https://timesmachine.nytimes.com/timesmachine/1953/08/30
/84420931.html?pageNumber=78.

Rigo, C., and Saroglou, V. "Religiosity and Sexual Behavior: Tense Relationships and Underlying Affects and Cognitions in Samples of Christian
and Muslim Traditions." *Archive for the Psychology of Religion* 40, nos.
2–3 (2018): 176–201.

Seper, F. "*Persona humana:* Declaration on Certain Questions Concerning Sexual Ethics," Delivered in Rome, December 29, 1975, at the Sacred
Congregation for the Doctrine of the Faith.

Southern Poverty Law Center. "Radical Traditional Catholicism."
2021. https://www.splcenter.org/fighting-hate/extremist-files/ideology
/radical-traditional-catholicism.

Speed, D., and Cragun, R. T. "Response to "Masturbation: Scientific Evidence and Islam's View." *Journal of Religion and Health* 60
(2021): 1668–1671.

Sprankle, E., Danielson, S., Lyng, T., and Severud, M. "Satanic Sexuality:
Understanding Satanism as a Diversity Issue for Sex and Relationship
Therapists." *Sexual and Relationship Therapy* 37, no. 3 (2021): 395–409.

Stephenson, K. "'It Is Done'—Latter-Day Saint Sex Therapist Natasha Helfer Is Ousted from the Church." *Salt Lake Tribune*, April 21,
2021. https://www.sltrib.com/religion/2021/04/21/lds-sex-therapist
-natasha/.

Sumer, Z. H. "Gender, Religiosity, Sexual Activity, Sexual Knowledge, and
Attitudes toward Controversial Aspects of Sexuality." *Journal of Religion
and Health* 54, no. 6 (2015): 2033–2044.

Zatat, N. "This Christian Author Says Female Masturbation 'Opens A
Portal to Hell.'" *Indy100*, April 13, 2016. https://www.indy100.com/news

/this-christian-author-says-female-masturbation-opens-a-portal-to-hell
-7295281.

Chapter 3
Semen, the Magical Elixir: Retention, Culture-Bound Syndromes, and
Insecure Incels

Aboul-Enein, B. H., Bernstein, J., and Ross, M. W. "Evidence for Masturbation and Prostate Cancer Risk: Do We Have a Verdict?" *Sexual Medicine Review* 4 (2016): 229–234.

American Psychiatric Association. *The Diagnostic and Statistical Manual of Mental Disorders,* 5th edition, text revision. Washington, DC: American Psychiatric Association, 2022.

Ayad, B. M., Horst, G. V., and Plessis, S. S. D. "Revisiting the Relationship between the Ejaculatory Abstinence Period and Semen Characteristics." *International Journal of Fertility & Sterility* 11 (2018): 238–246.

Carani, C., Granata, A. R., Rochira, V., Caffagni, G., Aranda, C., and Antunez, P. "Sex Steroids and Sexual Desire in a Man with a Novel Mutation of Aromatase Gene and Hypogonadism." *Psychoneuroendocrinology* 30 (2005): 413–417.

Carosa, E., Martini, P., Brandetti, F., Di Stasi, S. M., Lombardo, F., and Lenzi, A. "Type V Phosphodiesterase Inhibitor Treatments for Erectile Dysfunction Increase Testosterone Levels." *Clinical Endocrinology* 61 (2004): 382–386.

Castellini, G., Fanni, E., Corona, G., Maseroli, E., Ricca, V., and Maggi, M. "Psychological, Relational, and Biological Correlates of Ego-Dystonic Masturbation in a Clinical Setting." *Sexual Medicine* 4 (2016): e156–e165.

Chakrabarti, N., Chopra, V. K., and Sinha, V. K. "Masturbatory Guilt Leading to Severe Depression and Erectile Dysfunction." *Journal of Sex & Marital Therapy* 28 (2002): 285–287.

Chang, S. T. *The Tao of Sexology: The Book of Infinite Wisdom*. San Francisco: Tao Publishing, 1986.

Chughtai, B. "A Neglected Gland: A Review of Cowper's Gland." *International Journal of Andrology* 28, no. 2 (2005): 74–77.

Coleman, E. "Masturbation as a Means of Achieving Sexual Health." *Journal of Psychology & Human Sexuality* 14 (2003): 5–16.

Das, A. "Masturbation in the United States." *Journal of Sex & Marital Therapy* 33 (2007): 301–317.

Das, A., and Sawin, N. "Social Modulation or Hormonal Causation? Linkages of Testosterone with Sexual Activity and Relationship Quality in a Nationally Representative Longitudinal Sample of Older Adults." *Archives of Sexual Behavior* 45 (2016): 2101–2115.

De Jonge, C., LaFromboise, M., Bosmans, E., Ombelet, W., Cox, A., and Nijs, M. "Influence of the Abstinence Period on Human Sperm Quality." *Fertility and Sterility* 82 (2004): 57–65.

Escasa, M. J., Casey, J. F., and Gray, P. B. "Salivary Testosterone Levels in Men at a U.S. Sex Club." *Archives of Sexual Behavior* 40 (2011): 921–926.

Exton, M. S., Krüger, T. H. C., Bursch, N., Haake, P., Knapp, W., and Schedlowski, M. "Endocrine Response to Masturbation-Induced Orgasm in Healthy Men Following a 3-Week Sexual Abstinence." *World Journal of Urology* 19 (2001): 377–382.

Fuss, J., Bindila, L., Wiedemann, K., Auer, M. K., Briken, P., and Biedermann, S. V. "Masturbation to Orgasm Stimulates the Release of the Endocannabinoid 2-Arachidonoylglycerol in Humans." *Journal of Sexual Medicine* 14, no. 11 (2017): 1372–1379.

Georgiadis, J. R., and Kringelbach, M. L. "The Human Sexual Response Cycle: Brain Imaging Evidence Linking Sex to Other Pleasures." *Progress in Neurobiology* 98, no. 1 (2012): 49–81.

REFERENCES

Graham, S. *A Lecture to Young Men on Chastity. Intended Also for the Serious Consideration of Parents and Guardians.* Boston: Light and Sterns, 1837.

Hanson, B. M., Aston, K. I., Jenkins, T. G., Carrell, D. T., and Hotaling, J. M. "The Impact of Ejaculatory Abstinence on Semen Analysis Parameters: A Systematic Review." *Journal of Assisted Reproduction and Genetics* 35 (2018): 213–220.

Hartmann, M. "The Totalizing Meritocracy of Heterosex: Subjectivity in NoFap." *Sexualities* 24 (2020): 409–430.

Holstege, G., Georgiadis, J. R., Paans, A. M., Meiners, L. C., van der Graaf, F. H., and Reinders, A. S. "Brain Activation during Human Male Ejaculation." *Journal of Neuroscience* 23, no. 27 (2003): 9185–9193.

Isenmann, E., Schumann, M., Notbohm, H. L., Flenker, U., and Zimmer, P. "Hormonal Response after Masturbation in Young Healthy Men—A Randomized Controlled Cross-Over Pilot Study." *Basic and Clinical Andrology* 31, no. 1 (2021): 32.

Jiang, M., Jiang, X., Zou, Q., and Shen, J. "A Research on the Relationship between Ejaculation and Serum Testosterone Level in Men." *Journal of Zhejiang University of Science* 4 (2003): 236–240.

Komisaruk, B. R., Beyer-Flores, C., and Whipple, B. *The Science of Orgasm.* Baltimore: Johns Hopkins University Press, 2006.

Kruger, T. H., Haake, P., Chereath, D., Knapp, W., Janssen, O. E., Exton, M. S., and Hartmann, U. "Specificity of the Neuroendocrine Response to Orgasm during Sexual Arousal in Men." *Journal of Endocrinology* 177, no. 1 (2003): 57–64.

Maheshwari, P. N., Tillu, N. D., and Shah, U. S. "Extreme Self-Mutilation Due to 'Dhat' Syndrome." *Indian Journal of Urology* 38 (2022): 243–244.

Mascherek, A., Reidick, M. C., Gallinat, J., and Kühn, S. "Is Ejaculation Frequency in Men Related to General and Mental Health? Looking Back and Looking Forward." *Frontiers in Psychology* 12 (2021): 1–13.

Odent, M. *The Scientification of Love*. London: Free Association Books, 1999.

Owen, D. H. and Katz, D. F. "A Review of the Physical and Chemical Properties of Human Semen and the Formulation of a Semen Simulant." *Journal of Andrology* 26 (2005): 459–469.

Prakash, O., Kar, S. K., and Sathyanarayana Rao, T. S. "Indian Story on Semen Loss and Related Dhat Syndrome." *Indian Journal of Psychiatry* 56, no. 4 (2014): 377–382.

Prause, N., and Binnie, J. "Iatrogenic Effects of Reboot/NoFap on Public Health: A Preregistered Survey Study." *Sexualities* (2023). https://doi.org/10.1177/13634607231157070

Reid, D. P. *The Tao of Health, Sex, and Longevity: A Modern Practical Guide to the Ancient Way*. New York: Atria Books, 1989.

Rider, J. R., Wilson, K. M., Sinnott, J. A., Kelly, R. S., Mucci, L. A., and Giovannucci, E. L. "Ejaculation Frequency and Risk of Prostate Cancer: Updated Results with an Additional Decade of Follow-Up." *European Urology* 70 (2016): 974–982.

Sokolow, J. A. *Eros and Modernization: Sylvester Graham, Health Reform, and the Origins of Victorian Sexuality in America*. Cranbury, NJ: Associated University Presses, 1983.

Sørensen, M. B., Bergdahl, I. A., Hjøllund, N. H., Bonde, J. P., Stoltenberg, M., and Ernst, E. "Zinc, Magnesium and Calcium in Human Seminal Fluid: Relations to Other Semen Parameters and Fertility." *Molecular Human Reproduction* 5, no. 4 (1999): 331–337.

Sumathipala, A., Siribaddana, S. H., and Bhugra, D. "Culture-Bound Syndromes: The Story of Dhat Syndrome." *British Journal of Psychiatry* 184 (2004): 200–209.

Udina, M., Foulon, H., Valdes, M., Bhattacharyya, S., and Martin-Santos, R. "Dhat Syndrome: A Systematic Review." *Psychosomatics* 54, no. 3 (2013): 212–218.

REFERENCES

Van Anders, S. M., and Watson, N. V. "Social Neuroendocrinology: Effects of Social Contexts and Behaviors on Sex Steroids in Humans." *Human Nature* 17 (2006): 212–237.

Zhang, H. H., and Rose, K. *Who Can Ride the Dragon? An Exploration of the Cultural Roots of Traditional Chinese Medicine.* Brookline, MA: Paradigm Publications, 1999.

Zimmer, F., and Imhoff, R. "Abstinence from Masturbation and Hypersexuality." *Archives of Sexual Behavior* 49 (2020): 1333–1343.

Zukerman, Z., Weiss, D. B. and Orvieto, R. "Does Pre-Ejaculatory Penile Secretion Originating from Cowper's Gland Contain Sperm?" *Journal of Assisted Reproduction and Genetics* 20 (2003): 157–159.

Chapter 4
Addicted to Self-Diagnosing: Masturbation Addiction, Moral Incongruence, and Expensive 12 Steps

Carnes, P. J. *Out of the Shadows: Understanding Sexual Addiction.* Minneapolis, MN: CompCare Publications, 1983.

Crosby, J. M., and Twohig, M. P. "Acceptance and Commitment Therapy for Problematic Internet Pornography Use: A Randomized Trial." *Behavior Therapy* 47, no. 3 (2016): 355–366.

Dickenson, J. A., Gleason, N., Coleman, E., and Miner, M. H. "Prevalence of Distress Associated with Difficulty Controlling Sexual Urges, Feelings, and Behaviors in the United States." *JAMA Network Open* 1, no. 7 (2018): e184468.

Elist, J. J. "Masturbation Addiction." Dr. Elist, n.d. https://www.drelist.com/blog/masturbation-addiction/.

Grubbs, J. B., Grant, J. T., and Engelman, J. "Self-Identification as a Pornography Addict: Examining the Roles of Pornography Use, Religiousness, and Moral Incongruence." *Sexual Addiction & Compulsivity* 25, no. 4 (2019): 269–292.

Grubbs, J. B., Hoagland, K. C., Lee, B. N., Grant, J. T., Davison, P., Reid, R. C., and Kraus, S. W. "Sexual Addiction 25 Years On: A Systematic and Methodological Review of Empirical Literature and an Agenda for Future Research." *Clinical Psychology Review* 82 (2020): 101925.

Grubbs, J. B., Kraus, S. W., and Perry, S. L. "Self-Reported Addiction to Pornography in a Nationally Representative Sample: The Roles of Use Habits, Religiousness, and Moral Incongruence." *Journal of Behavioral Addictions* 8, no. 1 (2019): 88–93.

Grubbs, J. B., Kraus, S. W., Perry, S. L., Lewczuk, K., and Gola, M. "Moral Incongruence and Compulsive Sexual Behavior: Results from Cross-Sectional Interactions and Parallel Growth Curve Analyses." *Journal of Abnormal Psychology* 129, no. 3 (2020): 266–278.

Grubbs, J. B., Lee, B. N., Hoagland, K. C., Kraus, S. W., and Perry, S. L. "Addiction or Transgression? Moral Incongruence and Self-Reported Problematic Pornography Use in a Nationally Representative Sample." *Clinical Psychological Science* 8, no. 5 (2020): 936–946.

Grubbs, J. B., Perry, S. L., Wilt, J. A., and Reid, R. C. "Pornography Problems Due to Moral Incongruence: An Integrative Model with a Systematic Review and Meta-Analysis." *Archives of Sexual Behavior* 48 (2019): 397–415.

Hallberg, J., Kaldo, V., Arver, S., Dhejne, C., Jokinen, J., and Oberg, K. G. "A Randomized Controlled Study of Group-Administered Cognitive Behavioral Therapy for Hypersexual Disorder in Men." *Journal of Sexual Medicine* 16, no. 5 (2019): 733–745.

James, S. D. "Hypersexuality Disorder in Line to Become a Mental Diagnosis." ABC News, October 11, 2012. https://abcnews.go.com/Health/hypersexuality-disorder-line-mental-diagnosis/story?id=17455671.

Kafka, M. P. "Hypersexual Disorder: A Proposed Diagnosis for DSM-V." *Archives of Sexual Behavior* 39, no. 2 (2010): 377–400.

Kafka, M. P. "What Happened to Hypersexual Disorder?" *Archives of Sexual Behavior* 43, no. 7 (2014): 1259–1261.

Lewczuk, K., Szmyd, J., Skorko, M., and Gola, M. "Treatment Seeking for Problematic Pornography Use Among Women." *Journal of Behavioral Addictions* 6, no. 4 (2017): 445–456.

Ley, D. J. *The Myth of Sex Addiction*. Lanham, MD: Rowan and Littlefield, 2012.

Ley, D. J., Prause, N., and Finn, P. "The Emperor Has No Clothes: A Review of the 'Pornography Addiction' Model." *Current Sexual Health Reports* 6, no. 2 (2014): 94–105.

Rissel, C., Richters, J., Visser, R. O. de, McKee, A., Yeung, A., and Caruana, T. "A Profile of Pornography Users in Australia: Findings from the Second Australian Study of Health and Relationships." *Journal of Sex Research* 54, no. 2 (2017): 227–240.

Rush, B. *Medical Inquiries and Observations, upon the Diseases of the Mind*. Philadelphia: Kimber and Richardson, 1812.

Wainberg, M. L., Muench, F., Morgenstern, J., Hollander, E., Irwin, T. W., Parsons, J. T., Allen, A., and O'Leary, A. "A Double-Blind Study of Citalopram versus Placebo in the Treatment of Compulsive Sexual Behaviors in Gay and Bisexual Men." *Journal of Clinical Psychiatry* 67, no. 12 (2006): 1968–1973.

Walton, M. T. "Incongruence as a Variable Feature of Problematic Sexual Behaviors in an Online Sample of Self-Reported 'Sex Addiction.'" *Archives of Sexual Behavior* 48, no. 2 (2019): 443–447.

Wan, M., Finlayson, R., and Rowles, A. "Sexual Dependency Treatment Outcome Study." *Sexual Addiction & Compulsivity* 7, no. 3 (2000): 177–196.

Chapter 5
This Is Your Brain on Porn Illiteracy: Fight the New Drug, Porn Research, and Antisemitic Conspiracy Theories

Allen, S. "'Porn Kills Love': Mormons' Anti-Smut Crusade." *Daily Beast*, October 20, 2015. https://www.thedailybeast.com/porn-kills-love -mormons-anti-smut-crusade.

Brand, M., Snagowski, J., Laier, C., and Maderwald, S. "Ventral Striatum Activity When Watching Preferred Pornographic Pictures Is Correlated with Symptoms of Internet Pornography Addiction." *NeuroImage* 129, no. 1 (2016): 224–232.

Bridges, A. J., and Morokoff, P. J. "Sexual Media Use and Relational Satisfaction in Heterosexual Couples." *Personal Relationships* 18, no. 4 (2011): 562–585.

Campbell, L., and Kohut, T. "The Use and Effects of Pornography in Romantic Relationships." *Current Opinion in Psychology* 13 (2017): 6–10.

Cole, S. "The Crusade against PornHub Is Going to Get Someone Killed." *Vice,* April 13, 2021. https://www.vice.com/en/article/n7bj9w/anti-porn -extremism-pornhub-traffickinghub-exodus-cry-ncose.

Dickson, E. J. "How a New Meme Exposes the Far-Right Roots of #NoNutNovember." *Rolling Stone,* November 8, 2019. https://www .rollingstone.com/culture/ culture-features/coomer-meme-no-nut -november-nofap-908676/amp/.

Ferguson, C. J., and Hartley, R. D. "The Pleasure Is Momentary . . . The Expense Damnable? The Influence of Pornography on Rape and Sexual Assault." *Aggression and Violent Behavior* 14 (2009): 323–329.

Ferguson, C. J., and Hartley, R. D. "Pornography and Sexual Aggression: Can Meta-Analysis Find a Link?" *Trauma, Violence, & Abuse* 23, no. 1 (2022): 278–287.

Foubert, J. D., Brosi, M. W., and Bannon, R. S. "Pornography Viewing among Fraternity Men: Effects on Bystander Intervention, Rape Myth Acceptance and Behavioral Intent to Commit Sexual Assault." *Sexual Addiction & Compulsivity* 18, no. 4 (2011): 212–231.

Gola, M., Wordecha, M., Sescousse, G., et al. "Can Pornography Be Addictive? An fMRI Study of Men Seeking Treatment for Problematic Pornography Use." *Neuropsychopharmacology* 42 (2017): 2021–2031.

REFERENCES

Grubbs, J. B., and Gola, M. "Is Pornography Use Related to Erectile Functioning? Results from Cross-Sectional and Latent Growth Curve Analyses." *Journal of Sexual Medicine* 16, no. 1 (2019): 111–125.

Grubbs, J. B., and Perry, S. L. "Moral Incongruence and Pornography Use: A Critical Review and Integration." *Journal of Sex Research* 56, no. 1 (2019): 29–37.

Grubbs, J. B., Wright, P. J., Braden, A. L., Wilt, J. A., and Kraus, S. W. "Internet Pornography Use and Sexual Motivation: A Systematic Review and Integration." *Annals of the International Communication Association* 43, no. 2 (2019): 117–155.

Hay, M. "Why Science Has No Idea Whether Porn Is Good or Bad for You." *InsideHook,* September 15, 2020. https://www.insidehook.com /article/sex-and-dating/is-porn-good-or-bad.

Jacobs, T., Geysemans, B., Van Hal, G., Glazemakers, I., Fog-Poulsen, K., Vermandel, A., De Wachter, S., and De Win, G. "Associations between Online Pornography Consumption and Sexual Dysfunction in Young Men: Multivariate Analysis Based on an International Web-Based Survey." *JMIR Public Health Surveillance* 7, no. 10 (2021): e32542.

Jensen, R. "How Porn Makes Inequality Sexually Arousing." *Washington Post*, May 25, 2016. https://www.washingtonpost.com/news /in-theory/wp/2016/05/25/how-porn-makes-inequality-sexually -arousing/.

Kerl, K. "'Oppression by Orgasm': Pornography and Antisemitism in Far-Right Discourses in the United States since the 1970s." *Studies in American Jewish Literature* 39, no. 1 (2020): 117–138.

Kingston, D. A., Federoff, P., Firestone, P., Curry, S., and Bradford, J. M. "Pornography Use and Sexual Aggression: The Impact of Frequency and Type of Pornography Use on Recidivism among Sexual Offenders." *Aggressive Behavior* 34 (2008): 341–351.

REFERENCES

Kohut, T., Baer, J. L., and Watts, B. "Is Pornography Really about 'Making Hate to Women'? Pornography Users Hold More Gender Egalitarian Attitudes Than Nonusers in a Representative American Sample." *Journal of Sex Research* 53, no. 1 (2016): 1–11.

Kohut, T., Balzarini, R. N., Fisher, W. A., Grubbs, J. B., Campbell, L., and Prause, N. "Surveying Pornography Use: A Shaky Science Resting on Poor Measurement Foundations." *Journal of Sex Research* 57, no. 6 (2020): 722–742.

Komlenac, N., and Hochleitner, M. "Associations between Pornography Consumption, Sexual Flexibility, and Sexual Functioning among Austrian Adults." *Archives of Sexual Behavior* 51, no. 2 (2022): 1323–1336.

Kühn, S., and Gallinat, J. "Brain Structure and Functional Connectivity Associated with Pornography Consumption: The Brain on Porn." *JAMA Psychiatry* 71, no. 7 (2014): 827–834.

Kuznia, R. "Among Some Hate Groups, Porn Is Viewed as a Conspiracy." *New York Times,* June 17, 2019. https://www.nytimes.com/2019/06/07/us/hate-groups-porn-conspiracy.html.

Landripet, I., and Štulhofer, A. "Is Pornography Use Associated with Sexual Difficulties and Dysfunctions among Younger Heterosexual Men?" *Journal of Sexual Medicine* 12, no. 5 (2015): 1136–1139.

Litsou, K., Byron, P., McKee, A., and Ingham, R. "Learning from Pornography: Results of a Mixed Methods Systematic Review." *Sex Education* 21, no. 2 (2021): 236–252.

Love, T., Laier, C., Brand, M., Hatch, L., and Hajela, R. "Neuroscience of Internet Pornography Addiction: A Review and Update." *Behavioral Sciences* 5, no. 3 (2015): 388–433.

Mancini, C., Reckdenwald, A., and Beauregard, E. "Pornographic Exposure over the Life Course and the Severity of Sexual Offenses: Imitation and Cathartic Effects." *Journal of Criminal Justice* 40, no. 1 (2012): 21–30.

Mellor, E., and Duff, S. "The Use of Pornography and the Relationship between Pornography Exposure and Sexual Offending in

Males: A Systematic Review." *Aggression and Violent Behavior* 46 (2019): 116–126.

Muusses, L. D., Kerkhof, P., and Finkenauer, C. "Internet Pornography and Relationship Quality: A Longitudinal Study of within and between Partner Effects of Adjustment, Sexual Satisfaction and Sexually Explicit Internet Material among Newly-Weds." *Computers in Human Behavior* 45 (2015): 77–84.

Owen, T. "Leaked Chats Reveal Fascist Group Patriot Front Shames Members about Their Porn, Junk Food Habits." *Vice,* January 26, 2022. https://www.vice.com/en/article/ 5dg5gn/patriot-front-leaked-chats -porn-habits.

Perry, S. L. "Is the Link between Pornography Use and Relational Happiness Really More about Masturbation? Results from Two National Surveys." *Journal of Sex Research* 57, no. 1 (2020): 64–76.

Perry, S. L., and Whitehead, A. L. "Only Bad for Believers? Religion, Pornography Use, and Sexual Satisfaction among American Men." *Journal of Sex Research* 56, no. 1 (2019): 50–61.

Pine, L. N. N. *The Family in the Third Reich, 1933–1945*. Doctoral dissertation, University of London, 1996. Campus repository. http://etheses .lse.ac.uk/1410/1/U084457.pdf.

Poulsen, F. O., Busby, D. M., and Galovan, A. M. "Pornography Use: Who Uses It and How It Is Associated with Couple Outcomes." *Journal of Sex Research* 50, no. 1 (2013): 72–83.

Prause, N. "Porn Is for Masturbation." *Archives of Sexual Behavior* 48, no. 8 (2019): 2271–2277.

Romboy, D. "Utah Becomes First State to Declare Pornography a Public Health Crisis." *Desert News,* April 19, 2016. https://www.deseret.com /2016/4/19/20586970/utah-becomes-first-state-to-declare-pornography -a-public-health-crisis.

Short, M. B., Black, L., Smith, A. H., Wetterneck, C. T., and Wells, D. E. "A Review of Internet Pornography Use Research: Methodology and

Content from the Past 10 Years." *Cyberpsychology, Behavior, and Social Networking* 15, no. 1 (2012): 13–23.

Southern Poverty Law Center. "David Duke," n.d. https://www.splcenter .org/fighting-hate/extremist-files/individual/david-duke.

Staley, C., and Prause, N. "Erotica Viewing Effects on Intimate Relationships and Self/Partner Evaluations." *Archives of Sexual Behavior* 42 (2013): 615–624.

Szymanski, D. M., Feltman, C. E., and Dunn, T. L. "Male Partners' Perceived Pornography Use and Women's Relational and Psychological Health: The Roles of Trust, Attitudes, and Investment." *Sex Roles* 73 (2015): 187–199.

Voon, V., Mole, T. B., Banca, P., et al. "Neural Correlates of Sexual Cue Reactivity in Individuals with and without Compulsive Sexual Behaviors." *PLoS ONE* 9, no. 7 (2014): e102419.

Winer, S., and Wootliff, R. "Jenna Jameson Flogs David Duke over Claim Jews Rule Porn." *Times of Israel*, December 5, 2016. https://www .timesofisrael.com/jenna-jameson-flogs-david-duke-over-claim-jews -rule-porn/.

Wright, P. J., Tokunaga, R. S., and Kraus, A. "A Meta-Analysis of Pornography Consumption and Actual Acts of Sexual Aggression in General Population Studies." *Journal of Communication* 66, no. 1 (2016): 183–205.

Wright, P. J., Tokunaga, R. S., Kraus, A., and Klann, E. "Pornography Consumption and Satisfaction: A Meta-Analysis." *Human Communication Research* 43, no. 3 (2017): 315–343.

Chapter 6
Know Thyself: Sex Therapy, Learning to Come, and Masturbation Explorers

Abdel-Hamid, E. L., Naggar, E. A., and El Gilany, A. H. "Assessment of as-Needed Use of Pharmacotherapy and the Pause-Squeeze Technique in Premature Ejaculation." *International Journal of Impotence Research* 13, no. 1 (2001): 41–45.

Barbach, L. G. *For Yourself: The Fulfillment of Female Sexuality*. New York: Doubleday, 1975.

Baxendale, E., Roche, K., and Stephens, S. "An Examination of Autoerotic Asphyxiation in a Community Sample." *Canadian Journal of Human Sexuality* 28, no. 3 (2019): 292–303.

Bering, J. "So Close, and Yet So Far Away: The Contorted History of Autofellatio." *Slate,* August 8, 2011. https://slate.com/technology/2011 /08/autofellatio-the-contorted-history.html.

Binik, Y. M., and Hall, K. S. K. *Principles and Practice of Sex Therapy,* 5th ed. New York: Guilford Press, 2014.

Both, S., and Laan, E. "Directed Masturbation: A Treatment of Female Orgasmic Disorder." In *Cognitive Behavior Therapy: Applying Empirically Supported Techniques in Your Practice,* edited by W. T. O'Donohue and J. E. Fisher, 158–166. Hoboken, NJ: John Wiley and Sons, 2008

Cooper, K., Martyn-St James, M., Kaltenthaler, E., Dickinson, K., Cantrell, A., Wylie, K., Frodsham, L., and Hood, C. "Behavioral Therapies for Management of Premature Ejaculation: A Systematic Review." *Sexual Medicine* 3, no. 3 (2015): 174–188.

Dodson, B. *Liberating Masturbation: A Meditation on Self Love*. Self-published, 1978.

———. *Sex for One: The Joy of Self-Loving*. New York: Three Rivers Press, 1996.

Heiman, J. R. "Psychologic Treatments for Female Sexual Dysfunction: Are They Effective and Do We Need Them?" *Archives of Sexual Behavior* 31 (2002): 445–450.

Heiman, J. R., LoPiccolo, L., and LoPiccolo, J. *Becoming Orgasmic: A Sexual Growth Program for Women*. Hoboken, NJ: Prentice-Hall, 1976.

Jern, P. "Evaluation of a Behavioral Treatment Intervention for Premature Ejaculation Using a Handheld Stimulating Device." *Journal of Sex and Marital Therapy* 40 (2014): 358–366.

Kahn, E., and Lion, E. G. "A Clinical Note on a Self-Fellator." *American Journal of Psychiatry* 95 (1938): 131–133.

Kinsey, A., Pomeroy, W., and Martin, C. *Sexual Behavior in the Human Male*. Philadelphia: Saunders, 1948.

Laan, E., Rellini, A. H., and Barnes, T. "Standard Operating Procedures for Female Orgasmic Disorder: Consensus of the International Society for Sexual Medicine." *Journal of Sexual Medicine* 10 (2013): 74–82.

Lehmiller, J. J. *Tell Me What You Want: The Science of Sexual Desire and How It Can Help You Improve Your Sex Life*. New York: Hachette, 2018.

LoPiccolo, J., and Lobitz, W. C. "The Role of Masturbation in the Treatment of Orgasmic Dysfunction." *Archives of Sexual Behavior* 2, no. 2 (1972): 163–171.

Marcus, B. "Changes in a Woman's Sexual Experience and Expectations Following the Introduction of Electric Vibrator Assistance." *Journal of Sexual Medicine* 8 (2010): 3398–3498.

Masters, W. H., and Johnson, V. E. *Human Sexual Inadequacy*. Boston: Little, Brown, 1970.

Oguzhanoglu, N. K., Ozdel, O., and Aybek, Z. "The Efficacy of Fluoxetine and a Stop-Start Technique in the Treatment of Premature Ejaculation and Anxiety." *Journal of Clinical Psychopharmacology* 25 (2005): 192–194.

Riley, A. J., and Riley, E. J. "A Controlled Study to Evaluate Directed Masturbation in the Management of Primary Orgasmic Failure in Women." *British Journal of Psychiatry* 133 (1978): 404–409.

Rowland, D., McMahon, C. G., Abdo, C., Chen, J., Jannini, E., Waldinger, M. D., and Ahn, T. Y. "Disorders of Orgasm and Ejaculation in Men." *Journal of Sexual Medicine* 7, no. 4 (2010): 1668–1686.

Sauvageau, A., and Racette, S. "Autoerotic Deaths in the Literature from 1954 to 2004: A Review." *Journal of Forensic Sciences* 51, no. 1 (2006): 140–146.

Stahl, M. "The Psychedelic Science of 'Gooning'—Or Masturbating into a Trance." *Mel Magazine,* November 20, 2020. https://melmagazine.com /en-us/story/gooning-porn-how-to-goon-reddit-edging-masturbation.

Tourjée, D. "A Guide to Muffing: The Hidden Way to Finger Trans Women." *Vice,* October 12, 2017. https://www.vice.com/en/article/59dx w3/a-guide-to-muffing-the-hidden-way-to-finger-trans-women.

Chapter 7
Dildo Control: Vibrators, Sex Dolls, and Foreign Body Insertions

Adam and Eve Inc. v. Greg Abbott, Texas Attorney General. United States Court of Appeals for the Fifth Circuit. No. 06-51104 (2007).

Addiego, F., Belzer Jr., E. G., Comolli, J., Moger, W., Perry, J. D., and Whipple, B. "Female Ejaculation: A Case Study." *Journal of Sex Research* 17, no. 1 (1981): 13–21.

Amos, J. "Ancient Phallus Unearthed in Cave." BBC News, July 25, 2005. http://news.bbc.co.uk/1/hi/sci/tech/4713323.stm.

Bedi, N., El-Husseiny, T., Buchholz, N., and Masood, J. "'Putting Lead in Your Pencil': Self-Insertion of an Unusual Urethral Foreign Body for Sexual Gratification." *JRSM Short Reports* 1, no. 2 (2010): 18.

Comella, L. *Vibrator Nation: How Feminist Sex-Toy Stories Changed the Business of Pleasure.* Durham, NC: Duke University Press, 2017.

———. "20 Years Later, How the 'Sex and the City' Vibrator Episode Created a Lasting Buzz." *Forbes,* August 7, 2018. https://www.forbes.com

REFERENCES

/sites/lynncomella/2018/08/07/20-years-later-how-the-sex-and-the-city
-vibrator-episode-created-a-lasting-buzz/?sh=3129873d649b.

Davis, C., Blank, J., Lin, H., et al. "Characteristics of Vibrator Use among
Women." *Journal of Sex Research* 33, no. 4 (1996): 313–320.

Ferguson, A. *The Sex Doll: A History*. Jefferson, NC: McFarland and
Company, 2014.

Gräfenberg, E. "The Role of the Urethra in Female Orgasm." *International
Journal of Sexology* 3, no. 3 (1950): 145–148.

Harper, C. A., Lievesley, R., and Wanless, K. "Exploring the Psychological Characteristics and Risk-Related Cognitions of Individuals Who Own Sex Dolls." *Journal of Sex Research* (2022). https://doi.org
/10.1080/00224499.2022.2031848.

Hejna, P., Zátopková, L., and Janík, M. "Rectal Explosion: A Strange Case
of Autoerotic Death." *International Journal of Legal Medicine* 135, no. 1
(2021): 307–312.

Herbenick, D., Bowling, J., Dodge, B., et al. "Sexual Diversity in the
United States: Results from a Nationally Representative Probability
Sample of Adult Women and Men." *PLoS One* 12, no. 7 (2017): 1–23.

Herbenick, D., Reece, M., Sanders, S., et al. "Prevalence and Characteristics of Vibrator Use by Women in the United States: Results from
a Nationally Representative Study." *Journal of Sexual Medicine* 6, no. 7
(2009): 1857–1866.

Herbenick, D., Reece, M., Schick, V., et al. "Beliefs about Women's Vibrator Use: Results from a Nationally Representative Probability Sample."
Journal of Sex and Marital Therapy 37, no. 5 (2011): 329–345.

Hines, T. M. "The G-spot: A Modern Gynecologic Myth." *Clinical Opinion* 185, no. 2 (2001): 359–362.

Ladas, A. K., Whipple, B., and Perry, J. D. *The G Spot and Other Recent
Discoveries about Human Sexuality*. New York: Dell Publishing, 1982.

REFERENCES

Levin, R. J. "Prostate-Induced Orgasms: A Concise Review Illustrated with a Highly Relevant Case Study." *Clinical Anatomy* 31 (2018): 81–85.

Lieberman, H. "Selling Sex Toys: Marketing and the Meaning of Vibrators in Early Twentieth-Century America." *Enterprise and Society* 17, no. 2 (2016): 393–433.

————. *Buzz: A Stimulating History of the Sex Toy.* New York: Pegasus Books, 2017.

Lieberman, H., and Schatzberg, E. "A Failure of Academic Quality Control: The Technology of Orgasm." *Journal of Positive Sexuality* 4, no. 2 (2018): 24–47.

Linbecker, M., Pottek, T., Hinck, D., Schotte, U., Langfeld, N., and Wagner, W. "Urinary Retention with Ruptured Fornix Caused by a Maggot: An Autoerotic Accident." *The Urologist (Der Urologe)* 44, no. 6 (2005): 674–677.

Lister, K. *A Curious History of Sex.* London: Unbound Publishing, 2020.

Packard, F. R. "An Analysis of Two Hundred and Twenty-One Cases of Foreign Body Introduced into the Male Bladder Per Urethram, with Report of a Recent Case." *Annals of Surgery* 25, no. 5 (1897): 568–599.

Pafs, J. "A Sexual Superpower or a Shame? Women's Diverging Experiences of Squirting/Female Ejaculation in Sweden." *Sexualities* 26, nos. 1–2 (2023): 180–194.

Pastor, Z., and Chmel, R. "Differential Diagnostics of Female 'Sexual' Fluids: A Narrative Review." *International Urogynecology Journal* 29, no. 5 (2017): 621–629.

Smiley, O. "A Glass Tumbler in the Rectum." *Journal of the American Medical Association* 72, no. 18 (1919): 1285.

Unruh, B. T., Nejad, S. H., and Stern, T. A. "Insertion of Foreign Bodies (Polyembolokoilamania): Underpinnings and Management Strategies." *Primary Care Companion to CNS Disorders* 14, no. 1 (2012): 1–26.

Valverde, S. *The Modern Sex Doll Owner: A Descriptive Analysis*. Master's thesis, California Polytechnic State University, 2012.

Vieira-Baptista, P., Lima-Silva, J., Preti, M., Xavier, J., Vendeira, P., and Stockdale, C. K. "G-spot: Fact or Fiction? A Systematic Review." *Sexual Medicine* 9, no. 5 (2021): 100435.

Waraich, N. G., Hudson, J. S., and Iftikhar, S. Y. "Vibrator-Induced Fatal Rectal Perforation." *New Zealand Medical Journal* 120, no. 1260 (2007): U2685.

Waskul, D., and Anklan, M. "'Best Invention, Second to the Dishwasher': Vibrators and Sexual Pleasure." *Sexualities* 23, nos. 5–6 (2020): 849–875.

Webber v. State. State of Texas Court of Criminal Appeals. No. 03-99-00225-CR, 2000.

Weissert, W., and Biesecker, M. "Ted Cruz Defended Texas Ban on the Sale of Sex Toys in State." Associated Press, April 15, 2016. https://apnews.com/article/lifestyle-texas-ted-cruz-campaign-2016-toys-28d236513f534d5385a3d51360e5cbf5.

Wood, R. *Consumer Sexualities: Women and Sex Shopping*. Milton Park, UK: Routledge, 2018.

Chapter 8
Manual Labor: Peep Shows, Camming, and Communal Cumming

Allen, M. "Giuliani Tells Sex-Based Shops That the End Is Drawing Near." *New York Times*, July 20, 1988. https://www.nytimes.com/1998/07/20/nyregion/giuliani-tells-sex-based-shops-that-the-end-is-drawing-near.html.

Bleakley, P. "'500 Tokens to Go Private': Camgirls, Cybersex and Feminist Entrepreneurship." *Sexuality and Culture* 18, no. 4 (2014): 892–910.

Cook, J. "Shaken from Her Pedestal: A Decade of New York City's Sex Industry under Siege." *City University of New York Law Review* 9, no. 1 (2005): 121–159.

Dickson, E. "Why Straight Men Are Joining Masturbation Clubs." *GQ,* February 26, 2019. https://www.gq.com/story/why-straight-men-are -joining-masturbation-clubs?verso=true.

Easterbrook-Smith, G. "OnlyFans as Gig-Economy Work: A Nexus of Precarity and Stigma." *Porn Studies* (2022). https://doi.org/10.1080 /23268743.2022.2096682

Frizzelle, C. "Seattle's Premier Men's Jack-Off Club Isn't Just for Gay Guys." *The Stranger,* June 19, 2019. https://www.thestranger.com/features /2019/06/19/40517670/ seattles-premier-mens-jack-off-club-isnt-just -for-gay-guys.

Jones, A. "For Black Models Scroll Down: Webcam Modeling and the Racialization of Erotic Labor." *Sexuality and Culture* 19, no. 4 (2015): 776–799.

———. "I Get Paid to Have Orgasms: Adult Webcam Models' Negotia- tion of Pleasure and Danger." *Signs: Journal of Women in Culture and Society* 42, no. 1 (2016): 227–256.

———. "The Pleasures of Fetishization: BBW Erotic Webcam Performers, Empowerment, and Pleasure." *Fat Studies* 8, no. 3 (2019): 279–298.

———. *Camming: Money, Power, and Pleasure in the Sex Work Industry.* New York: NYU Press, 2020.

Mustain, K. "Helping a Brother Out." *Slate,* December 13, 2018. https:// slate.com/human-interest/2018/12/bateworld-straight-gay-masturbation -meaning.html.

Richtel, M. "Intimacy on the Web, with a Crowd." *New York Times,* September 21, 2013. https://www.nytimes.com/2013/09/22/technology /intimacy-on-the-web-with-a-crowd.html.

Rosenberg, P. "Jack-Off Clubs: A Little History." Rain City Jacks Blog, September 9, 2015. https://www.raincityjacks.org/jack-off-clubs-a-little -history/.

Secret, M. "At Live Peep Shows, Getting a Glimpse of Times Square's Sordid Past." *New York Times,* October 16, 2014. https://www.nytimes .com/2014/10/17/ nyregion/the-live-peep-show-a-relic-of-a-bygone -times-square-endures.html.

Shane, Charlotte. "OnlyFans Isn't Just Porn ;)." *New York Times*, May 18, 2021. https://www.nytimes.com/2021/05/18/magazine/onlyfans-porn .html.

Sherman, J. "Why Some Guys Like Jerking Off Together." BuzzFeed News, July 28, 2018. https://www.buzzfeednews.com/article/jsherman /gay-men-mutual-masturbation-jack-off-groups.

Way, M. "Rain City Jacks Is Seattle's Premier Masturbation Club." *Vice,* September 10, 2015. https://www.vice.com/en/article/bnp5vd /rain-city-jacks-is-seattles-premier-masturbation-club.

Weber, B. "Disney Unveils Restored New Amsterdam Theater." *New York Times,* April 3, 1997. https://www.nytimes.com/1997/04/03/nyregion /disney-unveils-restored-new-amsterdam-theater.html.

Weitzer, R. "Sex Work: Paradigms and Politics." In *Sex for Sale: Prostitution, Pornography, and the Sex Industry,* 2nd ed., edited by Ronald Weitzer, 1–43. Milton Park, UK: Routledge, 2009.

Chapter 9
'Til Death Do Us Part: Successful Aging, Assisted Living, and Romantic Necrophilia

Abbey, E. C. *The Sexual System and Its Derangements.* Self-published pamphlet, 1875.

Archibald, C. "Sexuality, Dementia and Residential Care: Managers' Report and Response." *Health and Social Care in the Community* 6, no. 2 (1998): 95–101.

Beckman, N., Waern, M., Gustafson, D., and Skoog, I. "Secular Trends in Self-Reported Sexual Activity and Satisfaction in Swedish 70 Year Olds:

REFERENCES

Cross Sectional Survey of Four Populations, 1971–2001." *British Medical Journal* 337, no. 7662 (2008): 151–154.

Coleman, E. "Masturbation as a Means of Achieving Sexual Health." *Journal of Psychology and Human Sexuality* 14, nos. 2–3 (2003): 5–16.

Crowther, M. R., and Zeiss, A. M. "Cognitive-Behavior Therapy in Older Adults: A Case Involving Sexual Functioning." *Psychotherapy in Practice* 55, no. 8 (1999): 961–975.

DeLamater, J., and Koepsel, E. "Relationships and Sexual Expression in Later Life: A Biopsychosocial Perspective." *Sexual and Relationship Therapy* 30, no. 1 (2015): 37–59.

Ginsberg, T. B., Pomerantz, S. C., and Kramer-Feeley, V. "Sexuality in Older Adults: Behaviors and Preferences." *Age and Ageing* 34, no. 5 (2005): 475–480.

Haddad, P. M., and Benbow, S. M. "Sexual Problems Associated with Dementia: Part 1. Problems and Their Consequences." *International Journal of Geriatric Psychology* 8 (1993): 547–551.

———. "Sexual Problems Associated with Dementia: Part 2. Aetiology and Treatment." *International Journal of Geriatric Psychology* 8 (1993): 631–637.

Jordan, K. "Ernest Borgnine, 91, Reveals His Little Secret." *Boston Herald*, August 15, 2008. https://www.bostonherald.com/2008/08/15/ernest-borgnine-91-reveals-his-little-secret/.

Lee, D. M., Nazroo, J., O'Connor, D. B., Blake, M., and Pendleton, N. "Sexual Health and Well-Being among Older Men and Women in England: Findings from the English Longitudinal Study of Ageing." *Archives of Sexual Behavior* 45, no. 1 (2015): 133–144.

Lindau, S. T., Schumm, L. P., Laumann, E. O., Levinson, W., O'Muircheataigh, C. A., and Waite, L. J. "A Study of Sexuality and Health among Older Adults in the United States." *New England Journal of Medicine* 357, no. 8 (2007): 762–774.

REFERENCES

Mahieu, L., and Gastmans, C. "Older Residents' Perspectives on Aged Sexuality in Institutionalized Elderly Care: A Systematic Literature Review." *International Journal of Nursing Studies* 52, no. 12 (2015): 1891–1905.

Morrissey Stahl, K. A., Bower, K. L., Seponski, D. M., Lewis, D. C., Farnham, A. L., and Cava-Tadik, Y. "A Practitioner's Guide to End-of-Life Intimacy: Suggestions for Conceptualization and Intervention in Palliative Care." *Omega: Journal of Death and Dying* 77, no. 1 (2017): 15–35.

Roelofs, T. S. M., Luijkx, K. G., and Embregts, P. J. C. M. "Intimacy and Sexuality of Nursing Home Residents with Dementia: A Systematic Review." *International Psychogeriatrics* 27, no. 3 (2015): 367–384.

Štulhofer, A., Jurin, T., Graham, C., Enzlin, P., and Træen, B. "Sexual Well-Being in Older Men and Women: Construction and Validation of a Multi-Dimensional Measure in Four European Countries." *Journal of Happiness Studies* 20, no. 7 (2018): 2329–2350.

Sullivan, H. "Back to Life: UK Sex Doll Rental Firm Offers Widows Replicas of Their Dead Partners to Help Comfort Them." *Sun,* October 15, 2018. https://www.thesun.co.uk/news/7495264/sex-dolls-dead-partners-widows/.

Theobald, S. "How Is Betty Dodson, the Queen of Female Masturbation, Dying? Not Quietly." *Daily Beast,* August 27, 2020. https://www.thedailybeast.com/how-is-betty-dodson-the-queen-of-female-masturbation-dying-not-quietly?ref=scroll.

Tischer, B. "Masturbatory Behaviors among Older Adult Populations: A Literature Review." *Journal of Undergraduate Research at Minnesota State University, Mankato* 22, no. 2 (2022): 1–37.

Træen, B., Štulhofer, A., Janssen, E., Carvalheria, A. A., Hald, G. M., Lange, T., and Graham, C. "Sexual Activity and Sexual Satisfaction among Older Adults in Four European Countries." *Archives of Sexual Behavior* 48, no. 3 (2018): 815–829.

Villar, F., Celdran, M., Serrat, R., Faba, J., Genover, M., and Martinez, T. "Sexual Situations in Spanish Long-Term Care Facilities: Which Ones Cause the Most Discomfort to Staff?" *Sexuality Research and Social Policy* 16 (2018): 446–454.

Villar, F., Serrat, R., Celdran, M., and Faba, J. "Staff Attitudes and Reactions towards Residents' Masturbation in Spanish Long-Term Care Facilities." *Journal of Clinical Nursing* 25, nos. 5–6 (2016): 819–828.

Winston, A. "21 Grams Is a Sex Toy That Contains the Ashes of a Dead Partner." *Dezeen,* April 26, 2015. https://www.dezeen.com/2015/04/26/21-grams-sex-toy-contains-ashes-of-dead-partner-mark-sturkenboom/.

Wright, H., Jenks, R. A., and Lee, D. M. "Sexual Expression and Cognitive Function: Gender-Divergent Associations in Older Adults." *Archives of Sexual Behavior* 49, no. 1 (2019): 941–951.

Conclusion
Masturbation Liberation, Self-Care, and Happy Endings

Charara, S. "What the Goop Lab Gets Right (and Wrong) about Sex." *Wired,* January 25, 2020. https://www.wired.co.uk/article/goop-lab-sex-netflix.

Davies, W. *The Happiness Industry: How the Government and Big Business Sold Us Well-Being.* London: Verso Books, 2015.

Dickson, E. J. "We Fact-Checked Four of the Most Outrageous Claims in Gwyneth Paltrow's Netflix Show." *Rolling Stone,* January 29, 2020. https://www.rollingstone.com/culture/culture-features/gwyneth-paltrow-goop-lab-netflix-941830/amp/.

Gonzalez, I. "Why I Made Masturbation Part of My Self-Care Routine." *Oprah Daily,* February 7, 2019. https://www.oprahdaily.com/life/health/a26233305/masturbation-self-care-routine/.

Gunter, J. *The Vagina Bible: The Vulva and the Vagina: Separating the Myth from Medicine.* New York: Kensington, 2019.

Herbenick, D., Fu, T., Wasata, R., and Coleman, E. "Masturbation Prevalence, Frequency, Reasons, and Associations with Partnered Sex in the midst of the COVID-19 Pandemic: Findings from a U.S. Nationally Representative Survey." *Archives of Sexual Behavior* 52 (2023): 1317–1331.

Huff, A. "Liberation and Pleasure: Feminist Sex Shops and the Politics of Consumption." *Women's Studies* 47, no. 4 (2018): 427–446.

Michaeli, I. "Self-Care: An Act of Political Warfare or a Neoliberal Trap?" *Development* 60, nos. 1–2 (2017): 50–56.

Reynolds, M. "Think Goop Is Bad? It's Only the Tip of Netflix's Pseudoscience Iceberg." *Wired,* January 24, 2020. https://www.wired.co.uk /article/the-goop-lab-netflix-review.

Wang, A. B. "Gwyneth Paltrow's Goop Touted the 'Benefits' of Putting a Jade Egg in Your Vagina. Now It Must Pay." *Washington Post,* September 5, 2018. https://www.washingtonpost.com/health/2018/09/05 /gwyneth-paltrows-goop-touted-benefits-putting-jade-egg-your-vagina -now-it-must-pay/.

Williams, D. "The Roots of the Garden." *Journal of Sex Research* 27, no. 3 (1990): 461–466.

Anti–Masturbation Crusaders

For centuries, people have made it their life's work to prevent others from masturbating. Whether motivated by divinity, ignorance, or hatred, these anti-masturbation crusaders share a common goal of eradicating self-pleasure. And this shared agenda makes for some strange bedfellows. Priests, politicians, physicians, Taoists, radical feminists, and white supremacists are ideologically joined in their quest to make you feel guilty for touching yourself. So, if you find yourself on this list, look at your company and reconsider your life choices.

Dr. Emery Abbey (nineteenth-century American physician and author of *The Sexual Systems and Its Derangements*)

Greg Abbott (governor of Texas)

Pope Benedict XVI (pope: 2005–2013)

Shmuley Boteach (author of *Kosher Sex*)

Robert Bowers (antisemite and mass shooter)

Anders Behring Breivik (white nationalist and mass murderer)

Lori Carlin (Travis County, Texas, sheriff's deputy)

Dr. Patrick Carnes ("sex addiction" specialist)

Stephen Chang (author of *The Tao of Sexology*)

Bill Clinton (forty-second president of the United States)

Ted Cruz (US senator from Texas)

Dr. Gail Dines (professor and radical feminist)

Bob Dornan (former US representative from California)

David Duke (white supremacist)

Andrea Dworkin (radical feminist)

Michael Eisner (former CEO of Disney)

Nick Fuentes (white nationalist)

Dwight Gibbons (inventor of spiked penile rings)

Rudy Giuliani (former mayor of New York City)

Sylvester Graham (reverend and author of *A Lecture to Young Men on Chastity*)

Dr. Sayed Shahabuddin Hoseini (research associate)

Eliezer ben Hurcanus (first-century CE rabbi)

Dr. Robert Jensen (emeritus professor of journalism)

Charles Jones (Travis County, Texas, sheriff's deputy)

Dr. Martin Kafka (associate professor of psychiatry)

Dr. John Harvey Kellogg (nineteenth-century American physician and author of *Plain Facts for Old and Young*)

Ronald Lawler (priest in the Pittsburgh diocese)

Dr. Trish Leigh (certified brain health coach)

Pope Leo IX (pope: 1049–1054)

Mack Major (Christian author)

Bruce McConkie (Mormon apostle)

Makko Musagara (Christian minister from Nigeria)

Clay Olsen (founder of Fight the New Drug)

Dr. Frank Orland (psychoanalyst)

Candace Owens (conservative commentator)

Dr. Drew Pinsky (physician and host of *Sex Rehab*)

Daniel Reid (author of *The Tao of Health, Sex, and Longevity*)

Dr. Benjamin Rush (nineteenth-century American physician)

Dr. Samuel-Auguste Tissot (eighteenth-century Swiss physician)

Paul Joseph Watson (far-right commentator and conspiracy theorist)

Masturbation Liberators

Fortunately, the list of masturbation liberators is longer than the list of anti-masturbation crusaders. This is a testament to the forward (albeit non-linear and slow) progress of the sexual liberation movement. Among those in the movement are psychologists, sociologists, public health professors, historians, activists, and even a rogue nun. If you find yourself on this list, congratulations; you are making excellent life choices.

Dr. Tariq Al Habib (clinical psychologist)

Michelle Anklan (social worker)

Dr. Lonnie Barbach (clinical psychologist)

Mira Bellweather (sex educator and trans rights activist)

Dr. Jesse Bering (psychologist and professor of science communication)

Joani Blank (sex educator and founder of Good Vibrations)

Ernest Borgnine (Academy Award–winning actor)

Brutal Sphincter (gore-grind metal band)

Samantha Cole (journalist)

Dr. Eli Coleman (former director of the Institute for Sexual and Gender Health)

Jennifer Cook (professor of law)

Dr. Ryan Cragun (professor of sociology)

Dr. Clive Davis (emeritus associate professor of psychology)

Ej Dickson (journalist)

Betty Dodson (sex educator and activist)

Dr. Joycelyn Elders (former US surgeon general)

Margaret Farley (Catholic nun)

Justine Ang Fonte (sex educator)

Dr. Allen Frances (professor emeritus of psychiatry)

Christopher Frizzelle (journalist)

Irena Gonzalez (journalist)

Dr. Joshua Grubbs (associate professor of psychology)

Marlene Hartmann (sociology research fellow)

Natasha Helfer (sex therapist)

Dr. Debby Herbenick (professor of public health)

Virginia Johnson (sex researcher)

Dr. Angela Jones (professor of sociology)

Jacq Jones (sex toy retailer)

Dr. Kristoff Kerl (postdoctoral fellow of history)

Dr. Alfred Kinsey (biology professor and sex researcher)

Dr. Taylor Kohut (psychology research associate)

Dr. Thomas Laqueur (emeritus professor of history)

Anton Szandor LaVey (founder of the Church of Satan)

Dr. Justin Lehmiller (social psychologist)

Dr. David Ley (clinical psychologist)

Dr. Hallie Lieberman (historian)

Dr. Kate Lister (historian)

Dr. Charles Lobitz (clinical psychologist)

Dr. Joseph LoPiccolo (clinical psychologist)

Dr. Jeno Martin (professor of reproductive health)

Dr. William Masters (gynecologist and sex researcher)

Dr. Israel Meizner (physician)

Dr. Kate Morrissey Stahl (clinical associate professor of social work)

Dr. Jessica Påfs (senior lecturer and researcher)

Dr. Samuel Perry (professor of sociology)

Dr. Nicole Prause (neuroscientist)

Carol Queen (sex educator)

Paul Rosenberg (founder of Rain City Jacks)

Carlin Ross (sex educator)

John Sherman (journalist)

Dr. David Speed (professor of psychology)

Annie Sprinkle (artist and activist)

Michael Stahl (journalist)

Jade Stanley (sex doll maker)

Mark Sturkenboom (sex toy designer)

Demi Sutra (porn performer)

Stephanie Theobald (journalist)

Dr. Bente Træen (professor of psychology)

Dr. Feliciano Villar (professor of psychology)

Dr. Dennis Waskul (professor of sociology)

Dawn Webber (sex toy retailer)

Dr. Ronald Weitzer (professor of sociology)

Dr. Ruth Westheimer (sex therapist)

Dr. Beverly Whipple (emeritus professor of nursing)

Dr. Andrew Whitehead (associate professor of sociology)

Dr. Michele Yang (associate professor of pediatrics-neurology)

The Pleasure of Language: Masturbation Slang

The terms *masturbation, masturbate,* and *masturbating* appear over 900 times throughout this book. To avoid too much repetition, I occasionally replaced *masturbation* with broader terms like *solo sex*, more euphemistic terms like *self-pleasure*, or the pathologizing terms of yore like *self-pollution, self-abuse,* and *the solitary vice.*

Largely absent, however, (aside from *DIY* in the title) are the dozens of slang terms for masturbation that developed in the English language over the centuries. Some of these slang terms are well-known and have their roots in popular literature and plays, whereas others were likely created by giggling teenagers on Reddit. Whatever their origin, I present to you a list of some of my favorites, and I challenge you to incorporate them into casual conversations, academic presentations, and school board meetings.

Auditioning the finger puppets

Badgering the witness

Bashing the bishop

Basting the ham

Boxing the Jesuit

Buffin' the muffin

Burping the baby

Camping at Crystal Lake

Celebrating Palm Sunday

Checking in at the Bates Motel

Chopping wood

Clock-working the orange

Conjuring Ophelia

Dancing the two-finger taco tango

Dating Pamela Handerson

Dialing the rotary phone

Diddling the fiddle

Discovering the Blair Witch

DJing at Club Bean

Doing a Meg Ryan

Dotting the i

Double clicking the mouse

Engaging in hand-to-gland combat

Exorcising Pazuzu

Feeding bologna to the Smurfs

Finding the old woman in the tub

Firing the surgeon general

Fist fighting the flamingo

Flicking the bean

Flogging the dolphin

Having traffic with thy self

Hitching a ride with Franklin

Hugging the hog

Inaugurating the worm

Googling oneself

Jackin' the beanstalk

Jerkin' the gherkin

Jilling off

Liquidating the inventory

Making fapple sauce

Making the bald man cry

Meeting with Rosie Palm

Milking the eel

Nulling the void

Paddling the pink canoe

Painting the picket fence

Paying at the turnpike

Playing the clitar

Pleading the fifth

Polishing the pearl

Pulling the pope

Punching the clown

Riding the unicycle

Robbing the zombie

Rubbing one out

Shucking the corn

Signing your name in the devil's book

Slamming the Spam

Slinging your jelly

Spanking the lemur

Stirring the mac and cheese

Strangling the babysitter

Stretching the pipe

Surfing the slit

Taking a trip to the Green Sea

Threatening the llama

Touching up one's lip gloss

Using Satan's typewriter

Varnishing the banister

Visiting the bat cave

Voting for oneself

Waxing the Buick

Whitewashing with Huck Finn

Wiggling the walrus

Working from home

Acknowledgments

From the conception of an idea to approving its final draft, I've spent over two years working on this book. The writing was often solitary, but the process relied on many others to see it through to its completion. And, for that, I wish to express sincere appreciation and gratitude:

To my agent, Michael Bourret, for being the first person in the publishing world to take a gamble on me, for advocating for me, and for promptly responding to my oft-neurotic emails to soothe my anxiety.

To my editor, Jessica Firger, for being immediately enthusiastic about this book the first day the proposal was sent to Union Square for consideration. You've challenged me to become a better writer, and your feedback has exponentially improved the quality of the book.

To my therapist for having to listen to my insecurities for the past two years and for challenging my maladaptive schemas, which allowed me to make progress on the writing.

To Lake Nokomis and Marilyn Manson's album *Holy Wood* for providing the environment and ambience in which the majority of this book was written.

To Howard Stern and Jerry Seinfeld for being my creative muses.

To Excedrin for managing my daily headaches.

To my family, especially my parents, for always showing me unconditional love and support. I appreciate how you've always expressed being proud of me and my accomplishments, and the difficulty it must be explaining to your friends what I do for a living. This book will make it more difficult.

To my cats, who can't read, but have appreciated my warm lap from my laptop and have provided me a lifetime worth of cuddles.

ACKNOWLEDGMENTS

And, most importantly, to my wife, who has championed this book from the beginning and who has always had my back. You're my best friend and my confidante. You understand me more than anyone ever has and never questioned my ability to succeed in this endeavor. For your unwavering support, empathy, and understanding, I love you.

Index

INDEX

INDEX

INDEX

Sex Addiction Screening Test (SAST), 79
Sex and the City (TV show), 135, 136
sex dolls, 149–150, 177–178
sex education, 19–20, 30–36, 113–122
Sex for One (Dodson), 114
Sex Rehab with Dr. (TV show), 75–76
sex therapy. *See* therapy
sex toys, 129–150
    dildos, 38, 129–132, 132n, 141, 178
    dolls, 149–150, 177–178
    female ejaculation, 140–144, 142n
    g-spots, 139–140, 141, 144–145, 144n
    history of, 38, 131–135, 132n
    legalization of, 129–131
    medical emergencies and, 145–148
    modern masturbatory
        technology, 148–149
    moral panic about, 150
    prostate milking and, 144–145
    vibrators, 114, 132–139, 133n, 141, 178
sexual addiction. *See* "addiction"
    to masturbation
sexuality education, 19–20, 30–36, 113–122
sexual sublimation, 91–92
The Sexual System and Its Derangements
    (Abbey), 167–168
sexual transmutation, 61–62
sex workers
    camming, 154–160
    discrimination and, 157–158
    live peep shows, 151–154
    shame. *See also* "addiction" to masturbation;
        religious beliefs
    jack-off clubs and, 163
    learning shame, 27–30
    moral incongruence and, 85–87, 98
    sex education for reducing, 31
    sex toy use and, 150
    sexual sublimation and, 91–92
Sherman, John, 163
Smiley, Orvall, 146
Solitary Sex (Laqueur), 12
Speed, David, 49
Sprinkle, Annie, 101, 175
squirting, 140–144, 142n
SSRI antidepressants, 120, 120n
Stahl, Michael, 121–122
Stanley, Jade, 177
stop-start technique, 118–121

stress management, 87–89, 185–186
Strick, Simon, 107
Sturkenboom, Mark, 178
Sutra, Demi, 154–155

Talmud, 46–47
Taoism, 61–65, 61n, 69–70
The Tao of Sex, Health, and Longevity
    (Reid), 63
The Tao of Sexology (Chang), 62
"teledildonics," 148–149
Tell Me What You Want
    (Lehmiller), 126–127
Temple of Pleasure, 113–114
testosterone, 67–68
Theobald, Stephanie, 175
therapy
    for "addiction" to masturbation,
        82–83, 89–94
    BodySex Workshops, 113–115, 174–175
    directed masturbation
        programs, 115–117
    for ejaculatory control, 117–122
toddler masturbation, 22–23, 26
Tomcat (Instagram handle), 64–65
Træen, Bente, 170

Utah Coalition Against Pornography, 96

vaginal eggs, 182, 183
vibrators, 114, 132–139, 133n, 141, 178
Villar, Feliciano, 172

Waskul, Dennis, 136–137
Watson, Paul Joseph, 105
Webber, Dawn, 129–130
Weitzer, Ronald, 155–156
wellness industry, 181–186
Westheimer, Ruth, 53
Whipple, Beverly, 139
Whitehead, Andrew, 97–98
white supremacists, 103–108
widowhood and grief, 175–179
Williams, Dell, 181
World Health Organization, 32

Yang, Michele, 22–23

zinc, 63, 69–70

About the Author

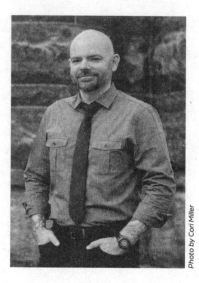

Photo by Cori Miller

Dr. Eric Sprankle is a professor of clinical psychology and codirector of the sexuality studies program at Minnesota State University, Mankato. He is also a licensed clinical psychologist and AASECT-certified sex therapist, affiliated with the Minnesota Sexual Health Institute. He received his doctorate in clinical psychology from Xavier University in 2009, completed a postdoctoral fellowship in sexual health at the University of Minnesota Medical School in 2011, and was awarded tenure in the Department of Psychology at Minnesota State University in 2017. When not defending himself against accusations of devil worship and witchcraft, he and his wife pass the time by staring at their three cats and actively avoiding small talk with neighbors.